Self-Management of Young People with Chronic Conditions

Jane N. T. Sattoe
AnneLoes van Staa • Sander R. Hilberink
Editors

Self-Management of Young People with Chronic Conditions

A Strength-Based Approach for Empowerment and Support

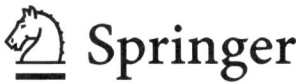

Editors
Jane N. T. Sattoe
Research Centre Innovations in Care
Rotterdam University of Applied Sciences
Rotterdam
The Netherlands

AnneLoes van Staa
Research Centre Innovations in Care
Rotterdam University of Applied Sciences
Rotterdam
The Netherlands

Sander R. Hilberink
Research Centre Innovations in Care
Rotterdam University of Applied Sciences
Rotterdam
The Netherlands

ISBN 978-3-030-64292-1   ISBN 978-3-030-64293-8   (eBook)
https://doi.org/10.1007/978-3-030-64293-8

This Springer imprint is published by the registered company Springer Nature Switzerland AG
The registered company address is: Gewerbestrasse 11, 6330 Cham, Switzerland

Contents

Marjolijn I. Bal, MSc graduated in psychology and is currently a PhD student. Her PhD thesis focuses on content and effectiveness of self-management and vocational rehabilitation interventions for young people with chronic physical conditions. She is also involved in research on the transition from secondary education to post-secondary education and vocational participation of young people with chronic physical conditions and autism.

Samuel M. Brotkin, MA has a BA in psychology from the University of North Carolina at Chapel Hill and an MA in clinical psychology from Duke University. His current research interests are focused on the health and well-being of adolescents and young adults living with pediatric chronic health conditions and their families, with a particular interest in cancer and cancer survivorship and examining the psychosocial, developmental, and health outcomes for this population.

Jodie Neukirch Elliott, MSW is a licensed clinical social worker. She has been involved in the planning and implementation of group support programs for adolescents with chronic health conditions since 2001. She is interested in both applying and studying the effects of positive youth development (PYD), leadership, and healthcare transition skills to group support programs. In addition to working clinically with youth with chronic health conditions and their families as a therapist, she is also involved in research in the utilization of peer health coaching to improve self-management and independence in adolescents and young adults who live with chronic health conditions.

Albert Farre, PhD is a social psychologist and applied health researcher based at the University of Dundee, UK. His research primarily focuses on adolescent and young adult health issues and broadly relates to psychosocial factors of health/illness and care behaviors, implementation science, and complex interventions, with a focus on understanding stakeholders' experiences to inform health policy and health service improvement. He also supervises masters and PhD research and teaches on implementing transitional care, health/care behaviors, and research methods across a range of health sciences programs.

Gemma Heath, PhD trained as a Health Psychologist at a specialist Children's Hospital in the UK. She conducts research into the lived experience of those with long-term and life-limiting health conditions, with a special interest in the role and experience of parents within young-person chronic condition management. She also works on the development, implementation, and evaluation of psychological interventions to improve health outcomes for young people with chronic conditions and their families.

Sander R. Hilberink, PhD is Applied Research Professor and trained as a clinical psychologist. He conducts research on transition to adulthood and lifespan care since 2006, with focus on empowerment, autonomy, and long-term consequences of childhood-onset chronic conditions. He is involved in a variety of healthcare innovations, addressing not only a better transfer to adult healthcare but also to improve citizenship while aging with lifelong disabilities.

Susan Kirk, PhD is Professor of Family and Child Health at the University of Manchester, UK. Her research interests relate to children's, young people's, and parents' experiences of childhood disability and long-term physical/mental illness and in understanding how support can be developed to meet their individual needs. Her research has examined issues relating to transition, self-management, and palliative care.

Alison R. S. Manning, MD obtained her medical degree from Drexel University and completed Triple Board combined residency and fellowship training in pediatrics, adult psychiatry, and child and adolescent psychiatry at Brown University. She is an Assistant Professor in the Division of Child and Family Mental Health at Duke University. She works on the Pediatric Psychiatry Consultation and Liaison service at Duke Children's Hospital serving patients with complex medical and psychiatric needs and is the medical director of Adolescents Transitioning to Leadership and Success, a peer mentorship group for children with chronic conditions at Duke. Dr. Manning is involved in research that focuses on harnessing the power of peer mentorship to improve adherence and outcomes for adolescents and young adults living with chronic conditions.

Gary Maslow, MD, MPH is a general pediatrician and child and adolescent psychiatrist with training in public health. He completed three residencies in pediatrics, psychiatry, and child and adolescent and psychiatry at Rhode Island Hospital/Brown University after attending Dartmouth Medical School. For the past 20 years he has been involved in developing peer support programs for youth with chronic illness including a program now at Duke called Adolescents Transitioning to Leadership and Success (ATLAS), a mentoring program with Duke University student mentors and high school aged mentees. Dr. Maslow leads a multidisciplinary team that includes social workers, psychologists, pediatricians, nurses, and child psychiatrists that is devoted to developing and disseminating peer support intervention for young adults with chronic illness and their families that utilize the Positive Youth Development framework.

Janet E. McDonagh, PhD, MD, MBBS is a practicing clinical consultant adolescent rheumatologist at Manchester University Hospitals Foundation Trusts as well as a Senior Lecturer in Adolescent Rheumatology at the Centre for Musculoskeletal Research, University of Manchester. She is involved in research in developmentally appropriate healthcare for young people including health transitions, vocational readiness, peer support in addition to work centered on chronic musculoskeletal pain during adolescence and young adulthood.

Linda J. Milnes, PhD, MPhil, RN is Associate Professor in Children and Young People's Nursing and trained as a general and pediatric nurse before becoming a lecturer and completing a National Institute for Health Research Doctoral Fellowship in 2010. Her areas of research interest relate to long-term conditions in childhood; children's, young people's, and parents'/carers' health beliefs; experiences of self-management and healthcare; exploring their support needs; and the development of complex self-management support interventions including an intervention to prepare young people for participation in consultations.

McLean D. Pollock, PhD, MSW is an Assistant Professor in the Department of Psychiatry and Behavioral Sciences at Duke University and a licensed clinical social worker and researcher in public health. Her research and clinical work focus on the psychosocial needs and strengths of individuals, caregivers, and families experiencing distress or complex care needs. Dr. Pollock oversees peer coaching and peer support programs for youth with special healthcare needs and their families, including the training and supervision of peer coaches, as well as the development, implementation, and evaluation of the coaching interventions.

Marij E. Roebroeck, PhD is associate professor at the Department of Rehabilitation Medicine of Erasmus University Medical Center and Rijndam Rehabilitation, Rotterdam. With her group she performs research on long-term consequences of childhood onset disabilities and on the effectiveness of age-appropriate interventions during the lifespan. She is leading national follow-up studies on youth and adolescents with cerebral palsy into adulthood and set up international consortia to develop core sets of outcomes for adults with cerebral palsy. She has recently extended her research focus to children with neurodisability at young age, connecting to the Pediatric Brain Center at the Sophia Children's Hospital of Erasmus University Medical Center.

Pepijn D. D. M. Roelofs, PhD is Assistant professor of work and health. His current research focusses on educating resilient nursing students and nursing graduates, in order to prevent work-related dropout from the profession. Other areas of interest are assessing work disability and rehabilitation programs for people with disabilities. He is an experienced researcher using mixed-method approaches in interdisciplinary research projects, collaborating with educational organizations, healthcare organizations, and multiple faculties.

Jane N. T. Sattoe, PhD graduated in health sciences. In 2015, she defended her PhD thesis "Growing up with a Chronic Condition: Challenges for Self-management and Self-management Support" about self-management of adolescents and young adults with chronic conditions. She is involved in research on transition to adulthood with a focus on self-management, transition to adult care, and mental health. She also works on the development, implementation, and evaluation of self-management interventions aiming to empower adolescents and young adults with chronic conditions.

Karen L. Shaw, PhD is a Research Psychologist at the University of Birmingham, UK. Her research focuses on transitional healthcare for children with long-term or life-threatening conditions. This includes transitions between services (e.g., from pediatric to adult healthcare) and transitions along the condition trajectory (e.g., from curative to end of life). As such, she has a special interest in how professionals and families can work together to plan care and improve services. She has been involved in transitional care research for the last 20 years and employs mixed methods that facilitate the user voice to be heard.

AnneLoes van Staa, PhD, MD, RN trained as a general and pediatric nurse before graduating both in medicine and cultural anthropology. In 2003, she was appointed professor of "Transitions in Care" at Rotterdam University of Applied Sciences. She defended her PhD thesis "On Your Own Feet" in 2012 about preferences and competencies of adolescents with chronic conditions in their transition to adulthood and to adult care. She is involved in quality improvement programs aimed at improving adolescent healthcare services and at empowering adolescents in self-management and autonomy. She also leads research programs into nurse-led self-management support of people with chronic conditions.

AnneLoes van Staa, Sander R. Hilberink,
and Jane N. T. Sattoe

1.1 Introduction: Chronic Health Conditions and Young People

Young people form an increasingly important group in current healthcare. Worldwide, at least 12% of adolescents grow up with a chronic disease, and most of them will reach adulthood [1]. Since national surveys often do not include mental, behavioral, or cognitive disorders, this percentage is probably an underestimation of the prevalence of chronic conditions in young people. Much depends on the definition used of a **chronic health condition**; see Box 1.1 for a non-categorical definition [2]. A non-categorical definition encompasses the consequences of conditions and reflects the child's functional status or ongoing use of medical services. Another example of such a definition is that of "Children with Special Health Care Needs" used in the USA: "those who have or are at increased risk for a chronic physical, developmental, behavioral, or emotional condition and who also require health and related services of a type or amount beyond that required by children generally" [3]. Using a non-categorical definition often yields higher prevalence rates up to 20–25% of all children. Nearly 20% of US children under 18 years of age have a special healthcare need [4]. Using health insurance data and a non-categorical definition comparable to the one presented in Box 1.1, a research institute based in the Netherlands established that in 2018, one in four Dutch children and young people (aged 0–25 years) suffered from a chronic health condition lasting longer than 3–6 months [5].

A chronic condition does not only include health issues linked to the illness young people suffer from, but also to adolescence and emerging adulthood in general, and to psychosocial problems generated by the interaction between the

A. van Staa (✉) · S. R. Hilberink · J. N. T. Sattoe
Research Center Innovations in Care, Rotterdam University of Applied Sciences,
Rotterdam, The Netherlands
e-mail: a.van.staa@hr.nl

© Springer Nature Switzerland AG 2021   1
J. N. T. Sattoe et al. (eds.), *Self-Management of Young People with Chronic
Conditions*, https://doi.org/10.1007/978-3-030-64293-8_1

Box 1.1: Definition of Chronic Health Conditions Originating in Childhood [2]
Chronic health conditions are defined as disorders that:
1. Have a biological, psychological, or cognitive basis;
2. Have lasted or are expected to last for at least 1 year; and
3. Produce one or more of the following sequelae:
    (a) Limitation of function, activities, or social role in comparison with healthy peers in the general areas of physical, cognitive, emotional, and social growth and development
    (b) Dependency on one of the following to compensate for or minimize limitation of function, activities, or social role: medications, special diet, medical technology or assistive device, personal assistance,
    (c) Need for medical care or related services, psychological services, or educational services over and above the usual for the child's age, or for special ongoing treatment, interventions, or accommodations at home or in school.

illness, the young person and his/her immediate environment. Young people who grow up with a chronic somatic condition and/or physical disability face various challenges during their transition to adulthood and to adult healthcare services. Becoming an adult represents a critical developmental stage for all young people as they experience multiple concurrent transitions including leaving high school and beginning post-secondary education, pursuing employment and getting a job, forming new social networks and personal relationships and moving out of parents' homes to independent living [6]. For young people with chronic health conditions, becoming an adult often proves extra challenging, because the adaptive tasks related to living with a chronic condition may clash with such developmental milestones. Finding a good balance and integrating these tasks in daily life is often referred to as **self-management**: the concept that is the central focus of this book. Effective self-management is considered essential for everyone living with chronic health problems, particularly for emerging adults with chronic health conditions [7]. Emerging adulthood involves a role shift in self-management responsibilities for them: ultimately, they are expected to take over the tasks and responsibilities for their self-management from their parents or caregivers. Taking up self-management is not an easy task; appropriate support can be of good use to young people growing up with a chronic condition and their parents alike. For this reason, there is an increasingly strong emphasis on the importance of self-management (support) in pediatric and young adult care, but to date, there is limited research on self-management promotion for young people [8–10].

This book will focus on the development and the support of self-management and empowerment of young people with chronic conditions. This volume, entitled *Self-Management of Young People with Chronic Conditions. A Strength-Based Approach for Empowerment and Support*, is unique in its broad view on self-management, i.e., it goes beyond medical management and focuses on young people achieving their full potential and a good quality of life. Furthermore, the book employs a positive youth development approach, focusing on empowerment and growth rather than problems or issues. Finally, it offers an overview of the state-of-the-art and evidence concerning self-management support for adolescents with various chronic conditions. Practical tools and instruments to help foster young people's self-management are also provided. As such, it is of benefit for all health-care professionals working in adolescent care, but also for researchers interested in this topic.

In this opening chapter, we now turn to discuss the major concepts employed in this book: healthcare transition, self-management (support), empowerment, auton-omy, and agency. Then, we present a short overview of the contents of the following chapters.

1.2   Healthcare Transition

The transition to adulthood of young people with chronic conditions is further complicated by the additional transition from pediatric services to the adult healthcare system. **Healthcare transition** is defined as the purposeful, coordi-nated, and planned movement of youth with chronic conditions from child-cen-tered to adult-oriented healthcare [11]. In the past decades, healthcare transition has become a recognized clinical need for young people with chronic long-term conditions as they approach the service termination deadline of the pediatric facility wherein they receive care. Betz and Coyne noticed that, over time, rec-ommendations for transitional care have evolved from putting emphasis on orga-nizational benchmarks and planning issues to more involved and comprehensive services [12]. This expansion of service deliverables includes self-management instruction, service coordination, referrals for community-based services, the emphasis of fostering independence, self-reliance, and the developmental com-petences associated with adulthood [13]. A person-centered and holistic approach is necessary to support young people in their transition. Professionals' attention should go beyond medical aspects and also address typical development and challenges of young people in their transition to adulthood. Developmentally appropriate care is essential to build young people's self-efficacy and to foster their transfer readiness.

An example of such a comprehensive transition services model is the On Your Own Feet Framework (Fig. 1.1) that addresses eight key elements of good transi-tional care, divided into three core categories: (1) interventions to improve the orga-nization of care; (2) interventions to stimulate independence and self-management of adolescents; and (3) collaboration with young people (and their families) and within the multidisciplinary team of professionals, working both in pediatric care and adult care [14]. These goals can be realized by using tools that focus on building skills for independent living and self-management (i.e., enhance self-efficacy). Chapter 8 discusses two examples of such plans that encourage young people to

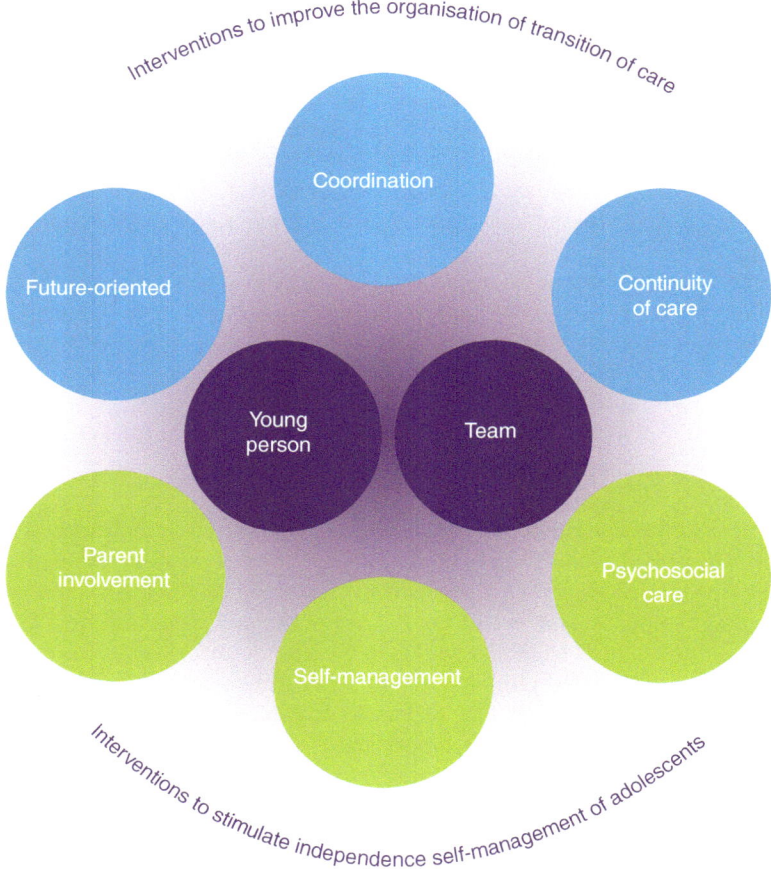

Fig. 1.1 The On Your Own Feet Framework for transitional care [14]

think about their future and to set their personal goals for gaining more autonomy in different life domains (e.g., healthcare, education, relationships, etc.).

There is a growing body of knowledge on healthcare transition. Recent textbooks (for example, [12, 15, 16]) have addressed transition from a wide range of professional (medical, nursing) perspectives or employed a systems approach. National guidelines and consensus statements have indicated which essential elements are part of good transitional care [17–20]. Numerous reviews have focused on the transition experiences of young people, parents, and healthcare professionals [21–24]. Recently, a multinational Delphi study indicated relevant outcomes [25], and the effective components of transitional care interventions have also been reviewed [26–28]. Still, the importance of fostering strategies to enable youth with chronic health conditions to work toward gradual self-management has not received as much attention [9]. Yet, self-management is key in successful transition to adult healthcare.

1.3   Self-Management

The concept of self-management is directly related to the challenges that children and young people with chronic health conditions and their parents or caretakers experience in their daily lives. While everyone is involved in self-care activities for themselves or others, such as getting dressed, providing nourishment, doing household chores, or looking after a sick family member, people living with chronic conditions have additional "work" to do in order to balance their health problems with daily life. This was first acknowledged by the sociologists Corbin and Strauss, who identified three types of "work" in managing a chronic condition in daily life: (1) illness-related work, i.e., dealing with the medical aspects of a chronic condition; (2) everyday life work, i.e., dealing with a condition in daily activities; and (3) biographical work, i.e., accepting change and giving a (new) meaning to life [29]. Lorig and Holman framed these three types of work as "medical (or behavioral) management", "role management" and "emotional (or identity) management," respectively [30]. This holistic view on self-management and the categorization of domains of self-management proposed by Lorig and Holman has been used in many studies (for example, [31–33]). In this book, we refer to these three domains related as follows: *medical management* (concerning the chronic condition and treatment thereof), *role management* (concerning social participation and social roles), and *emotional management* (concerning emotional well-being).

We view self-management as essential work that people with chronic conditions need to do in order to maintain the balance between managing their illness and their life. Self-management is therefore an empirical fact, inseparably and unavoidably connected to having a chronic condition [34]. It should not be regarded as an assignment given by healthcare professionals, but rather as an intrinsic part of living with a chronic condition. Self-management also implies that people with chronic conditions, young or old, determine to a large extent how they manage their condition on a daily basis in their own environment, without healthcare professionals present. Self-management is intrinsically linked to patient empowerment, and the acknowledgement of patients' right to self-determination.

Barlow and colleagues defined self-management as "the individual's ability to manage the symptoms, treatment, physical and psychosocial consequences and lifestyle changes inherent in living with a chronic condition" ([35], p. 178). The focus is on well-being and the ultimate goal of self-management is to maintain "a satisfactory quality of life" ([35], p. 178). We will use this broad definition in this book, because it acknowledges that living with a chronic condition requires not only managing symptoms and treatment, but also includes dealing with psychosocial consequences, social relations, and lifestyle changes that the condition incurs. With respect to the aim of self-management, Barlow and colleagues state that: "efficacious self-management encompasses the ability to monitor one's condition and to effect the cognitive, behavioral, and emotional responses necessary to maintain a satisfactory quality of life. Thus, a dynamic and continuous process of self-regulation is established" ([35], p. 178). In this view, patients' themselves define their goals to maintain optimal quality of life. This broad definition of self-management not only accounts for the dynamic life context of people with chronic conditions [35–40], but also empowers people living with chronic conditions: self-management is about taking (back) control over your health and life.

This view on self-management is not universal or undisputed. There is a lot of ambiguity surrounding the concept and there is no consensus about the definition or the purpose of self-management. There are different views on what efficacious self-management entails and what should be considered as the desirable outcomes of the process. Many healthcare professionals understand self-management to serve the purpose of improving clinical outcomes (e.g., by striving for optimal therapy adherence) [41, 42]. It reflects the medical viewpoint that considers healthcare professionals experts and focuses on optimal medical management of the chronic health condition. This view implies that healthcare professionals define what "good" self-management is and instruct patients what to do (or not do)—who are expected to follow these instructions. This narrow and directive view on self-management often conflicts with patient values and preferences, particularly in the case of chronic conditions where patients themselves have accumulated expert knowledge.

In other views, self-management refers to a complex and multidimensional construct (e.g., [8, 31, 43]). Strauss and Glaser described a chronic condition as a "negotiated reality" [44], emphasizing that people with chronic conditions are not always sick. Living with a chronic condition is described as an ongoing process of inner negotiation [45] and shifting between "illness-on-the-foreground" and "wellness-on-the-foreground" [46]. Studies showed that people with chronic conditions indeed switch between self-management patterns according to their changing needs and priorities in daily life [47], and emphasize that healthcare professionals should also switch between support styles to deliver tailored self-management support [48]. Thus, self-management is a dynamic process rather than a fixed reality, a static body of knowledge and skills [10]. It can be described as "a fluid, iterative process during which patients incorporate multidimensional strategies that meet their self-identified needs to cope with chronic disease within the context of their daily living" [8]. Self-management is learnt by doing as situations and conditions change and strategies need to be tested. As it is the result of many trial-and-error efforts, there is no fixed learning curve. This is challenging for young people who are beginning to take over responsibilities and learning to cope by themselves, as will be discussed in Chap. 3.

1.4   Supporting Self-Management

To become efficacious in self-management and establish a process of self-regulation, patients need problem-solving skills, need to understand how to monitor one's condition, have to make informed decisions, find and utilize resources, form partnership with their healthcare professionals, and take action [30]. Given these requirements, most patients will need self-management support from their family or friends and from professionals. While self-management is an individual's ability, it is by no means an ability developed outside the social context. The process of self-management is not done by the individual patient alone [49]. Some have therefore suggested to extend Barlow's definition. For example, Richard and Shea added that self-management is done "[…] in conjunction with family, community, and healthcare professionals […]" [50]. The importance of the social context and others who help with self-management is repeatedly underlined in the self-management literature, especially in case of young people growing up with chronic conditions [10, 51]. Some even argue that adult models of self-management in chronic conditions generally are not directly applicable to young people growing up with chronic conditions [7, 52–54]. In Chap. 3, we will elaborate on how the dynamic process of self-management of these young people differs from that of adults with chronic conditions. We explore specific frameworks of self-management (support) in young people with chronic conditions and review their (age-specific) self-management tasks, theories, interventions, and outcomes.

In this book, we embrace a person-centered view on self-management, and suggest that healthcare professionals take on a supportive role, based on lived experiences of young people and a strengths-based, positive view of the patients' abilities. The definition of self-management support we use is inspired by Bodenheimer et al. [55]: Self-management support is the support provided by healthcare professionals to patients and their families, so that patients can manage the physical, mental, and social consequences of their condition in daily life.

The process of delivering self-management support is often represented in the Five A's cycle model [56, 57]. The Five A's model is a framework with a counselling approach, entailing a series of sequential steps (Assess, Advise, Agree, Assist, and Arrange; Fig. 1.2). This approach emphasizes collaborative goal setting, patient skill building to overcome barriers, self-monitoring, personalized feedback, and systematic links to community recourses [56, 58].

Fig. 1.2 The 5-A's model describing the process of self-management support. (Adapted; based on Glasgow et al. [56])

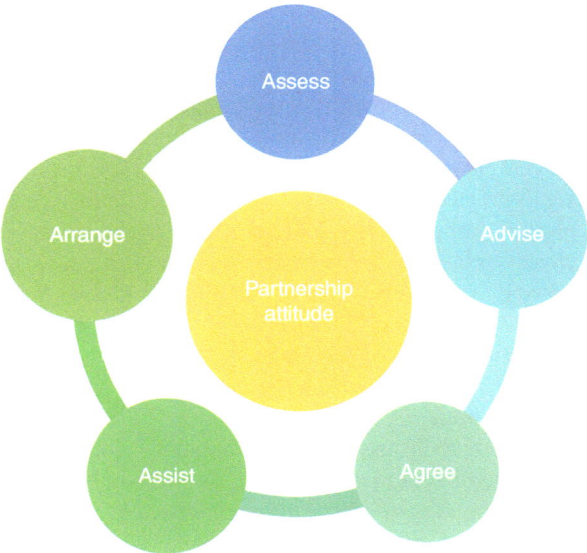

Increasing independence of youth cannot be seen separately from the role of parents as safety nets, and healthcare providers as enablers and collaborators [9]. Therefore, the roles in self-management support of parents and carers will receive attention in Chap. 6, while the challenges of the healthcare team in promoting self-management will be addressed in Chap. 5.

1.5   Empowerment, Autonomy, and Agency

A variety of definitions of **empowerment** have been coined. Following Gibson, empowerment has three key characteristics [59]. First, empowerment appears to be transactional, it requires meaningful relationships with others. Second, it is a developmental concept since it improves ones potential over time and depends on age-appropriate competences. In addition, empowerment appears to be dynamic as it results in changes in power. Third, empowerment is democratic because it contributes to social justice by redistributing power. As such it is a multidimensional concept that can been seen as both a process and an outcome [60]. 'Empowerment as process' refers to educating and encouraging young people to take control, to make decision themselves and to bear responsibility (i.e., the transactional and developmental concept) [61]. On the other hand, 'empowerment as outcome' often refers to being autonomous and competent to engage in adult roles (e.g., decision-making, self-advocacy) [60].

Empowerment has been associated with five domains, which might be helpful to measure it: (1) knowledge and understanding, (2) personal control, (3) identity, (4) shared decision-making, and (5) enabling others [62]. Taking these five domains into account, it becomes clear that empowerment not only aims at strengthening **autonomy** from a liberal point of view, but also targets identity-formation and interpersonal relationships, and promotes leadership. Liberal autonomy refers to independency, independent decision-making, and not being restricted by others. This is taking control and having agency. However, autonomy can also be seen from a relational perspective. Relational autonomy states that we all live in contexts and that everyone depends on others. So, interdependence is an important characteristic. Next to interdependence, another central aspect is personal development; where the self is created in relation to others. Thus, empowerment also stresses the importance of supporting identity-formation and engaging in healthy relationships. **Agency** closely relates to both perspectives on autonomy: having control over one's life, based on options between acceptable alternatives facilitating meaningful choices in life [63]. Agency does not mean that young people stand alone in their choices, it also refers to chose for support and building a significant network to be part of. Key is to shape life, including the needed support, according one's way of living and personal preferences [64].

Chapter 2 discusses the development, background, principles, and application of the Positive Youth Development. This strengths-based approach combines both liberal and relational perspectives on autonomy. In Chap. 8 two practical tools (self-management action plans) are presented to work with young people.

1.6   The Contents of This Book

The chapters in this book reflect various perspectives on the background, development, and promotion of self-management of young people with chronic conditions. The chapters explore self-management from the perspectives of youth, parents, and healthcare providers. The concept of self-management is examined in its broader context of development of young persons; whereby the importance of the adoption of a strength-based approach that empowers and supports young people is underlined. Furthermore, the book also reviews the existing evidence on support programs aimed at increasing self-management skills, improving relevant outcomes, and involving relevant others such as peers and parents in the process. Finally, the book offers more practical advice by discussing useful tools and interventions that healthcare professionals can apply in practice.

Chapters 2 and 3 further explore the underlying theories and the historical notions that support the development of self-management in young people. The authoring team headed by Alison Manning (Chap. 2) explores the Positive Youth Development approach: a theoretically based, developmental framework that is strengths-based, incorporates ecological assets, and has been applied and shown effective in at-risk youth, including those growing up with chronic health problems.

Chapter 3 builds on the discourse on self-management that was briefly presented in this chapter. Here, Jane Sattoe and AnneLoes van Staa explain the developmental context that affects the take-up of self-management in young people with chronic conditions, and the specific challenges they face when it comes to learning self-management skills. The chapter offers an overview of the adaptive tasks of growing up with a chronic health condition and concludes with a general typology of self-management interventions and of outcome measures.

The discussion of the evaluation of such self-management interventions and the role of healthcare professionals in delivering self-management support, is continued in Chaps. 4 and 5, albeit from different perspectives. In Chap. 4, the authoring team headed by Marjolijn Bal, reviews the effectiveness of self-management support by exploring which intervention components contribute to positive outcomes. The mode of delivery of self-management interventions (for example, individual or group-based), the type of interventionists (monodisciplinary or multidisciplinary), and the intended effect (improved adherence or coping, reduction of anxiety and depressive feelings, or increased life skills) are reviewed.

In Chap. 5, Janet McDonagh considers how health professionals, multidisciplinary teams, health systems, and the wider community can support and nurture self-management development during adolescence and young adulthood. Here, the focus is not only on the evidence, but also on understanding the barriers and facilitators in enabling young people to self-manage their health, their chronic condition, and its therapy, as well as learn to navigate the health systems providing their care.

Chapter 6 focuses on the important, but often overlooked role of parents and caregivers of young people with chronic conditions in the transition to adulthood. Karen Shaw and her team examine past and current thinking about parental involvement and show that parents are instrumental in promoting young people's health, well-being, and transitional readiness. They also highlight a number of ways to foster positive relationships with parents in adolescent care settings and challenge the prevailing view that young people are expected to manage their condition independently.

The role of peers is the subject of Chap. 7 written by Susan Kirk and Linda Milnes. This chapter examines definitions of peer support and its theoretical underpinnings, approaches and components. While there is no conclusive evidence for the effectiveness of peer support programs in improving young people's health and well-being, peer support is valued by young people. The authors also consider potential risks posed by peer support.

In Chap. 8, Jane Sattoe and colleagues discuss two practical tools (Skills for Growing Up and Ready Steady Go) to support the development of self-management and life skills for the successful transition to adulthood. Both tools facilitate the communication between youth, their parents and healthcare professionals, are age-appropriate and cover various life areas. Overall, youth and parents appreciate working with these communication tools. Healthcare professionals are generally positive about both tools, although implementation in clinical practice can be a challenge.

To ensure that self-management support programs are acceptable to and appropriate for young people, the authors of various chapters (Chaps. 3, 5, 6, 7, and 8) embrace the view that young people need to be involved in the development (co-creation) of such interventions and programs need to be theoretically informed. As youth depend on parents and healthcare providers for support in taking charge of their own health, parents and healthcare providers must work together to enable youth for self-management—employing a positive, strengths-based approach.

References

1. Sawyer SM, Drew S, Yeo MS, Britto MT. Adolescents with a chronic condition: challenges living, challenges treating. Lancet. 2007;369(9571):1481–9. https://doi.org/10.1016/S0140-6736(07)60370-5.
2. Stein RE, Bauman LJ, Westbrook LE, Coupey SM, Ireys HT. Framework for identifying children who have chronic conditions: the case for a new definition. J Pediatr. 1993;122(3):342–7. https://doi.org/10.1016/S0022-3476(05)83414-6.
3. McPherson M, Arango P, Fox H, Lauver C, McManus M, Newacheck PW, et al. A new definition of children with special health care needs. Pediatrics. 1998;102(1):137–9. https://doi.org/10.1542/peds.102.1.137.
4. Health Resources and Service Administration. Children with special health care needs. 2019. https://mchb.hrsa.gov//maternal-child-health-topics/children-and-youth-special-health-needs.
5. van Hal L, Tierolf B, van Rooijen M, van der Hoff M. Een actueel perspectief op kinderen en jongeren met een chronische aandoening in Nederland: omvang, samenstelling en participatie. [A recent perspective on children and youth with a chronic condition in the Netherlands: scope, composition and participation]. Utrecht: Verwey-Jonker Instituut; 2019.
6. Gorter J, Stewart D, Woodbury-Smith M. Youth in transition: care, health and development. Child Care Health Dev. 2011;37(6):757–63. https://doi.org/10.1111/j.1365-2214.2011.01336.x.

7. Modi AC, Pai AL, Hommel KA, Hood KK, Cortina S, Hilliard ME, et al. Pediatric self-management: a framework for research, practice, and policy. Pediatrics. 2012;129(2):e473–85. https://doi.org/10.1542/peds.2011-1635.

8. Miller WR, Lasiter S, Ellis RB, Buelow JM. Chronic disease self-management: a hybrid concept analysis. Nurs Outlook. 2015;63(2):154–61. https://doi.org/10.1016/j.outlook.2014.07.005.

9. Nguyen T, Henderson D, Stewart D, Hlyva O, Punthakee Z, Gorter J. You never transition alone! Exploring the experiences of youth with chronic health conditions, parents and healthcare providers on self-management. Child Care Health Dev. 2016;42(4):464–72. https://doi.org/10.1111/cch.12334.

10. Sattoe JNT. Growing up with a chronic condition: challenges for self-management and self-management support. Rotterdam: Erasmus University Rotterdam; 2015.

11. Blum RW, Garell D, Hodgman CH, Jorissen TW, Okinow NA, Orr DP, Slap GB. Transition from child-centered to adult health-care systems for adolescents with chronic conditions: a position paper of the Society for Adolescent Medicine. J Adolesc Health. 1993;14(7):570–6. https://doi.org/10.1016/1054-139X(93)90143-D.

12. Betz CL, Coyne IT. Transition from pediatric to adult healthcare services for adolescents and young adults with long-term conditions: an international perspective on nurses' roles and interventions. Cham: Springer; 2019. https://doi.org/10.1007/978-3-030-23384-6.

13. McDonagh JE, Farre A. Are we there yet? An update on transitional care in rheumatology. Arthritis Res Ther. 2018;20(1):1–3. https://doi.org/10.1186/s13075-017-1502-y.

14. van Staa AL, Peeters MAC, Sattoe JNT. On your own feet: a practical framework for improving transitional care and young people's self-management. In: Betz CL, Coyne I, editors. Transition from pediatric to adult healthcare services for young adults with long-term conditions. An international perspective on nurses' roles and interventions, Chapter 9. Cham: Springer International; 2020. p. 191–228. https://doi.org/10.1007/978-3-030-23384-6_9.

15. Hergenroeder AC, Wiemann CM. Health care transition: building a program for adolescents and young adults with chronic illness and disability. Cham: Springer; 2018. https://doi.org/10.1007/978-3-319-72868-1.

16. Wood D, Williams A, Koyle MA, Baird AD. Transitioning medical care: through adolescence to adulthood. Cham: Springer; 2019. https://doi.org/10.1007/978-3-030-05895-1.

17. Got Transition. The six core elements of health care. Transition. 2014;(2.0). http://www.got-transition.org.

18. Mazur A, Dembinski L, Schrier L, Hadjipanayis A, Michaud PA. European Academy of Paediatric consensus statement on successful transition from paediatric to adult care for adolescents with chronic conditions. Acta Paediatr. 2017;106(8):1354–7. https://doi.org/10.1111/apa.13901.

19. National Institute for Health Care Excellence. NICE guidelines [NG43] Transition from children's to adults' services for young people using health or social care services. 2016.

20. Surís J-C, Akré C. Key elements for, and indicators of, a successful transition: an international Delphi study. J Adolesc Health. 2015;56(6):612–8. https://doi.org/10.1016/j.jadohealth.2015.02.007.

21. Betz CL, Lobo ML, Nehring WM, Bui K. Voices not heard: a systematic review of adolescents' and emerging adults' perspectives of health care transition. Nurs Outlook. 2013;61(5):311–36. https://doi.org/10.1016/j.outlook.2013.01.008.

22. Fegran L, Hall EO, Uhrenfeldt L, Aagaard H, Ludvigsen MS. Adolescents' and young adults' transition experiences when transferring from paediatric to adult care: a qualitative metasynthesis. Int J Nurs Stud. 2014;51(1):123–35. https://doi.org/10.1016/j.ijnurstu.2013.02.001.

23. Heath G, Farre A, Shaw K. Parenting a child with chronic illness as they transition into adulthood: a systematic review and thematic synthesis of parents' experiences. Patient Educ Couns. 2017;100(1):76–92. https://doi.org/10.1016/j.pec.2016.08.011.

24. Nehring WM, Betz CL, Lobo ML. Uncharted territory: systematic review of providers' roles, understanding, and views pertaining to health care transition. J Pediatr Nurs. 2015;30(5):732–47. https://doi.org/10.1016/j.pedn.2015.05.030.

25. van den Brink G, van Gaalen MA, de Ridder L, van der Woude CJ, Escher JC. Health care transition outcomes in inflammatory bowel disease: a multinational Delphi study. J Crohn Col. 2019;13(9):1163–72. https://doi.org/10.1093/ecco-jcc/jjz044.
26. Campbell F, Biggs K, Aldiss SK, O'Neill PM, Clowes M, McDonagh J, et al. Transition of care for adolescents from paediatric services to adult health services. Cochrane Database Syst Rev. 2016;29(4):CD009794. https://doi.org/10.1002/14651858.CD009794.pub2.
27. Hart LC, Patel-Nguyen SV, Merkley MG, Jonas DE. An evidence map for interventions addressing transition from pediatric to adult care: a systematic review of systematic reviews. J Pediatr Nurs. 2019;48:18–34. https://doi.org/10.1016/j.pedn.2019.05.015.
28. Schultz AT, Smaldone A. Components of interventions that improve transitions to adult care for adolescents with type 1 diabetes. J Adolesc Health. 2017;60(2):133–46. https://doi.org/10.1016/j.jadohealth.2016.10.002.
29. Corbin JM, Strauss A. Unending work and care: managing chronic illness at home. San Fransisco, CA: Jossey-Bass; 1988.
30. Lorig KR, Holman HR. Self-management education: history, definition, outcomes, and mechanisms. Ann Behav Med. 2003;26(1):1–7. https://doi.org/10.1207/S15324796ABM2601_01.
31. Packer TL, Fracini A, Audulv Å, Alizadeh N, van Gaal BG, Warner G, Kephart G. What we know about the purpose, theoretical foundation, scope and dimensionality of existing self-management measurement tools: a scoping review. Patient Educ Couns. 2018;101(4):579–95. https://doi.org/10.1016/j.pec.2017.10.014.
32. Sattoe JNT, Bal MI, Roelofs PD, Bal R, Miedema HS, van Staa A. Self-management interventions for young people with chronic conditions: a systematic overview. Patient Educ Couns. 2015;98(6):704–15. https://doi.org/10.1016/j.pec.2015.03.004.
33. Van de Velde D, De Zutter F, Satink T, Costa U, Janquart S, Senn D, De Vriendt P. Delineating the concept of self-management in chronic conditions: a concept analysis. BMJ Open. 2019;9(7):e027775. https://doi.org/10.1136/bmjopen-2018-027775.
34. Grypdonck M. Zelfmanagement. [Self-management]. In: van den Brink R, Timmermans H, van Havers J, Veenendaal H, editors. Ruimte voor regie. Pioniers over zelfmanagement in de zorg. [Making room for taking control. Pioneers on self-management in healthcare]. Deventer/Utrecht: Kluwer/CBO; 2013.
35. Barlow J, Wright C, Sheasby J, Turner A, Hainsworth J. Self-management approaches for people with chronic conditions: a review. Patient Educ Couns. 2002;48(2):177–87. https://doi.org/10.1016/s0738-3991(02)00032-0.
36. Jones MC, MacGillivray S, Kroll T, Zohoor AR, Connaghan J. A thematic analysis of the conceptualisation of self-care, self-management and self-management support in the long-term conditions management literature. J Nurs Healthc Chronic Illn. 2011;3(3):174–85. https://doi.org/10.1111/j.1752-9824.2011.01096.x.
37. Jonsdottir H. Self-management programmes for people living with chronic obstructive pulmonary disease: a call for a reconceptualisation. J Clin Nurs. 2013;22(5–6):621–37. https://doi.org/10.1111/jocn.12100.
38. Koch T, Jenkin P, Kralik D. Chronic illness self-management: locating the 'self'. J Adv Nurs. 2004;48(5):484–92. https://doi.org/10.1111/j.1365-2648.2004.03237.x.
39. Schulman-Green D, Jaser S, Martin F, Alonzo A, Grey M, McCorkle R, et al. Processes of self-management in chronic illness. J Nurs Scholarsh. 2012;44(2):136–44. https://doi.org/10.1111/j.1547-5069.2012.01444.x.
40. Udlis KA. Self-management in chronic illness: concept and dimensional analysis. J Nurs Healthc Chronic Illn. 2011;3(2):130–9. https://doi.org/10.1111/j.1752-9824.2011.01085.x.
41. Bourbeau J. Disease-specific self-management programs in patients with advanced chronic obstructive pulmonary disease. Dis Manag Health Out. 2003;11(5):311–9. https://doi.org/10.2165/00115677-200311050-00004.
42. Coleman MT, Newton KS. Supporting self-management in patients with chronic illness. Am Fam Physician. 2005;72(8):1503–10.
43. Nightingale R, McHugh G, Kirk S, Swallow V. Supporting children and young people to assume responsibility from their parents for the self-management of their long-term condition:

an integrative review. Child Care Health Dev. 2019;45(2):175–88. https://doi.org/10.1111/cch.12645.

44. Strauss AL, Glaser BG. Chronic illness and the quality of life. St. Louis, MO: Mosby; 1975.
45. Audulv Å, Norbergh KG, Asplund K, Hörnsten Å. An ongoing process of inner negotiation–a Grounded Theory study of self-management among people living with chronic illness. J Nurs Healthc Chronic Illn. 2009;1(4):283–93. https://doi.org/10.1111/j.1752-9824.2009.01039.x.
46. Paterson BL. The shifting perspectives model of chronic illness. J Nurs Scholarsh. 2001;33(1):21–6. https://doi.org/10.1111/j.1547-5069.2001.00021.x.
47. Audulv Å. The over time development of chronic illness self-management patterns: a longitudinal qualitative study. BMC Public Health. 2013;13(1):452. https://doi.org/10.1186/1471-2458-13-452.
48. van Hooft SM, Dwarswaard J, Jedeloo S, Bal R, van Staa A. Four perspectives on self-management support by nurses for people with chronic conditions: a Q-methodological study. Int J Nurs Stud. 2015;52(1):157–66. https://doi.org/10.1016/j.ijnurstu.2014.07.004.
49. Dwarswaard J, Bakker EJ, van Staa A, Boeije HR. Self-management support from the perspective of patients with a chronic condition: a thematic synthesis of qualitative studies. Health Expect. 2016;19(2):194–208. https://doi.org/10.1111/hex.12346.
50. Richard AA, Shea K. Delineation of self-care and associated concepts. J Nurs Scholarsh. 2011;43(3):255–64. https://doi.org/10.1111/j.1547-5069.2011.01404.x.
51. Callery P, Coyne I. Supporting children and adolescents inclusion in decisions and self-management: what can help? Patient Educ Couns. 2019;102(4):605–6. https://doi.org/10.1016/j.pec.2019.03.003.
52. Kirk S. Transitions in the lives of young people with complex healthcare needs. Child Care Health Dev. 2008;34(5):567–75. https://doi.org/10.1111/j.1365-2214.2008.00862.x.
53. Lozano P, Houtrow A. Supporting self-management in children and adolescents with complex chronic conditions. Pediatrics. 2018;141(Suppl 3):S233–41. https://doi.org/10.1542/peds.2017-1284H.
54. Sawyer SM, Aroni RA. Self-management in adolescents with chronic illness. What does it mean and how can it be achieved? Med J Aust. 2005;183(8):405–9. https://doi.org/10.5694/j.1326-5377.2005.tb07103.x.
55. Bodenheimer T, Lorig K, Holman H, Grumbach K. Patient self-management of chronic disease in primary care. JAMA. 2002;288(19):2469–75.
56. Glasgow RE, Davis CL, Funnell MM, Beck A. Implementing practical interventions to support chronic illness self-management. Jt Comm J Qual Saf. 2003;29(11):563–74.
57. Whitlock EP, Orleans CT, Pender N, Allan J. Evaluating primary care behavioral counseling interventions: an evidence-based approach. Am J Prev Med. 2002;22(4):267–84.
58. Whitehead D. Health promotion and health education viewed as symbiotic paradigms: bridging the theory and practice gap between them. J Clin Nurs. 2003;12(6):796–805.
59. Gibson CH. A concept analysis of empowerment. J Adv Nurs. 1991;16(3):354–61. https://doi.org/10.1111/j.1365-2648.1991.tb01660.x.
60. Small N, Bower P, Chew-Graham CA, Whalley D, Protheroe J. Patient empowerment in long-term conditions: development and preliminary testing of a new measure. BMC Health Serv Res. 2013;13(1):263. https://doi.org/10.1186/1472-6963-13-263.
61. Mora MA, Sparud-Lundin C, Bratt E-L, Moons P. Empowering young persons during the transition to adulthood. In: Betz C, Coyne I, editors. Transition from pediatric to adult healthcare services for adolescents and young adults with long-term conditions. Cham: Springer; 2020. p. 19–46. https://doi.org/10.1007/978-3-030-23384-6_2.
62. Úcar Martínez X, Jiménez-Morales M, Soler Masó P, Trilla Bernet J. Exploring the conceptualization and research of empowerment in the field of youth. Int J Adolesc Youth. 2017;22(4):405–18. https://doi.org/10.1080/02673843.2016.1209120.
63. DeLoach C, Wilkins RD, Walker GW. Independent living: philosophy, process, and services. Baltimore, MD: University Park Press; 1983.
64. Hilberink SR, Cardol M. Agency in the twenty-first century: the emperor's new clothes. Disabil Soc. 2013;28(4):569–74. https://doi.org/10.1080/09687599.2013.790616.

Alison R. S. Manning, Jodie Neukirch Elliott,
Samuel M. Brotkin, Gary Maslow, and McLean D. Pollock

2.1 Introduction

As increasing numbers of adolescents and young adults (AYA) with childhood onset chronic conditions (COCC) are surviving into adulthood, the question of how to best support them has become increasingly important. These AYA with COCC deserve to not only grow up, but to thrive. This chapter focuses on Positive Youth Development (PYD) as a way of promoting positive outcomes for this population, such as social connectedness, enhanced confidence, community engagement, and increased prosocial behaviours. PYD is conceptualized as a developmental process, an approach to helping youth succeed, and the instances of youth programs that incorporate this theory. We begin by providing an overview of the societal context in which the PYD framework developed, including the shift to viewing youth as assets to be developed, rather than problems to be fixed. PYD posits that interactions between an individual and their environment are essential to promote developmental outcomes. We then explore a plethora of developmental theories that provide the basis for an empirically supported PYD approach, including Lerner and Lerner's 5Cs model of PYD, in which thriving is conceptualized as the growth of Competence, Confidence, Character, Connection, and Caring. Application of PYD principles to AYA with COCC is the focus of the remainder of the chapter.

The concept of AYA with COCC as a high-risk group is introduced, alongside research examining comparisons with peers without chronic conditions. While many AYA with COCC are eventually able to thrive, there may be marked differences in educational, vocational, and social outcomes [1–3]. For these reasons, applying a developmental, strengths-based approach to this population is crucial. We present research on PYD-based programming for AYA with COCC and bring

A. R. S. Manning (✉) · J. N. Elliott · S. M. Brotkin · G. Maslow · M. D. Pollock
Department of Psychiatry and Behavioral Sciences, Duke University School of Medicine,
Durham, NC, USA
e-mail: alison.manning@duke.edu

© Springer Nature Switzerland AG 2021
J. N. T. Sattoe et al. (eds.), *Self-Management of Young People with Chronic Conditions*, https://doi.org/10.1007/978-3-030-64293-8_2

attention to gaps in the literature. The "Big 3", including (1) opportunities for leadership, (2) emphasis on development of life skills and (3) sustained and supportive youth–adult relationships, are highlighted as essential components of youth programming to promote PYD in AYA [4]. Mentor relationships, opportunities for leadership, and summer camps for youth with COCC are opportune settings to integrate PYD components to enhance outcomes for AYA with COCC.

Recommendations on how to incorporate PYD components into both youth programming and interactions within the healthcare field are provided. While there is some research on PYD interventions for AYA with COCC, the need for rigorous evaluation continues; a variety of measures for examining PYD programming are suggested and reviewed. Increasing PYD has been linked to increases in competence and confidence, which can help empower young people to be more actively engaged in their own lives. AYA with COCC need to become independent in managing their healthcare, thus exposure to PYD components may aid in their development of life and healthcare transition skills. Since PYD focuses on the interaction between a person and their environment, and AYA with COCC often spend a significant amount of time in medical settings, understanding ways to encourage positive development and integrate it into healthcare may provide additional tools to promote successful adult development and improved health outcomes for this population.

2.2   The History and Evolution of Positive Youth Development

Positive Youth Development is a theory and an approach that is rooted in developmental psychology and conceptualizes youths as inherently capable of living positive and productive lives. In order to understand the PYD approach and model, it is important to appreciate how the field of youth development and youth development programs evolved. In the United States, in the late 1800s/early 1900s, children regularly worked at a young age, often in unsafe conditions. In the early 1900s, child labour and compulsory education laws began to gain support in the States [5], and youth development programs started providing educational and supportive services to children and adolescents. Many early programs were focused on providing safe places to help youth develop into productive, contributing members of society [6]. In 1938, Congress passed the Fair Labor Standards Act, which regulated child labour [7]. As more children were expected to attend school to a later age and were not allowed to work, the need for youth development programs increased. These early programs often included practical skills that youth could use in later life.

In the 1960s, there was a shift in societal thinking about youth, where the potential for self-destructive behaviour was emphasized, which led to a focus on "fixing" kids [8]. In response to the idea that youth were troubled and likely to engage in risky behaviours, programs began to focus on prevention of problems, such as drug use, drunk driving, gang affiliation and teenage pregnancy. This focus on risk behaviours and preventing delinquency fostered a negative lens through which to view youth. Rather than seeing adolescents' potential and ability to grow and contribute to society, programs and practices were developed to avoid or mitigate problems and negative outcomes. This "problem-youth tradition" contributed to viewing and characterizing adolescents as a problem to be fixed rather than as a resource to invest in and nurture [9].

By the 1980s, the idea that youth are typically *not* troubled and can be successful contributors to society began to gain traction. With this view of youth as having inherent positive qualities that could be utilized and harnessed, positive youth development theory began to solidify, leading to the growth of programs to help youth develop in positive, normative ways. This shift in how adolescents are portrayed resulted in a substantial increase in the use of strengths-based approaches to adolescent development by researchers, practitioners and policymakers. These efforts were derived from theories and philosophies of the positive youth development perspective, which underscored the importance of fostering the adolescent's strengths and capacity to thrive, rather than solely focusing on mitigating or eliminating risk behaviours [10].

In order to promote positive outcomes, the PYD framework also examines alignment between youths' strengths and the resources in their surroundings or community [11]. PYD scholars propose that all young people have strengths, and that their surrounding contexts, including other individuals, such as parents or mentors, and institutions, such as schools or programs, can provide them with resources that promote their development. These ecological factors have been positively associated with indicators of PYD and inversely related to risk behaviours [12]. When the strengths of youth are aligned with resources in the environment, positive outcomes and youth thriving are promoted.

There are several theories in the PYD tradition that have led to the current model of PYD. William Damon [9] wrote about adolescence as a time period where individuals start to explore their sense of purpose. Early research in the field indicated that motivation is developed when youth are able to identify their passion. This sense of purpose helps youth to have prosocial behaviours, commitment, achievement, and self-esteem; it also allows youth to identify moral values. Defined as, "a stable and generalized intention to accomplish something that is at once meaningful to the self and of consequence to the world beyond the self" [9], purpose is a combination of action-oriented goals, both short and long term, of one's desire to make a difference in the world and find meaning in his or her life [13]. Purpose is often viewed differently in adolescents and adults, and there may also be differences based on gender, socioeconomic, and cultural differences [13].

Peter Benson and the Search Institute examined developmental assets that young people should successfully develop, which formed the basis of the 5Cs as will be discussed. They identified 40 assets that serve as the building blocks for healthy adolescent development. These assets are organized into two broad categories— internal and external. Internal assets include commitment to learning, positive values, social competencies, and positive identity. External assets consist of family/ school/community supports, empowerment, boundaries and expectations, and constructive use of time [14]. There have been multiple studies that show the additive nature of these developmental assets, with young people with more assets faring better than those with fewer. Both genders show similar patterns, with higher levels of assets correlating with lower levels of risk behaviour and higher levels of indicators for thriving. Therefore, these assets have the potential to compensate for socio-economic status differences.

Between 2000 and 2002, the National Research Council and Institute of Medicine's Committee on Community-Level Programs for Youth met to determine the current state of youth programming in the United States and examined the social forces that led to changes in family/community life and expectations for young people [15]. They discovered several important factors negatively contributing to youth development, including weakening of community support, more parents working outside the home, greater exposure to violence in the media, and the extension of adolescence into the mid- to late-twenties. Since youth who have these unmet psychosocial needs are at higher risk for problem behaviours, they need enhanced supports. Thus, the committee determined, "young people need skills, knowledge, and a variety of other personal and social assets to function well during adolescence and adulthood" [15]. The universal themes identified were feeling competent, being connected socially, and having one's physical needs met. The committee recommended that community programs offer opportunities for youth to acquire developmental assets in positive settings as a means to reduce risk.

One such conduit of supporting youth development is through mentoring. Reed Larson added to the field of PYD by examining how mentoring relationships support development and youth agency. Based on Piaget's developmental theories, in which children are biologically wired to adapt to their environments [16], Larson [17] viewed young people as individuals who are "motivated and able to be constructive agents of their own development". Larson introduced the importance of this need to adapt and learn, which continues into adulthood. Individuals are more motivated to take on challenges when they have ownership over their actions, and, in turn, motivation supports learning and development. Larson found that mentoring interventions can work to change obstacles in daily life that may inhibit building developmental assets and that the input and guidance of the adult helps to support the youths' experience of agency, allowing the youth to navigate future situations independently. Larson's work contributes to the current model of PYD by exploring the positive effects of sustained youth–adult relationships.

The PYD framework has been further developed and studied by Lerner and Lerner and their 5Cs model of PYD [18]. The current formulation of the 5Cs model of PYD has evolved with contributions from the theorists mentioned above and the work of several other developmental scientists [19–21]. From 2000 to 2003, the current formulation of the 5Cs model emerged including Competence, Confidence, Connection, Character, and Caring (Table 2.1). The development of these components is aligned with Benson's earlier work on developmental assets, as all 40 assets can be mapped to at least one of the 5Cs. Competence is related to not only having the ability to perform a task well, but also to having a sense of related self-efficacy or perceiving that one can perform the job successfully. In terms of confidence, an individual must have an overall sense of self-worth. While individuals may be

Table 2.1 Definition of the 5Cs of positive youth development

Domain	Definition
Competence	Abilities/skills as well as a positive view of one's abilities/skills in domain specific areas, including social, academic, cognitive, and vocational
Confidence	An internal sense of overall positive self-worth and self-efficacy
Connection	Positive bonds with people and institutions that are reflected in bidirectional exchanges between the individual and peers, family, school, and community, in which both parties contribute to the relationship
Character	Respect for societal and cultural rules, possession of standards for correct behaviours, morality and integrity
Caring	A sense of sympathy and empathy for others

confident in certain abilities or actions, to fully meet this "C" a person has to have a positive self-image. Connection is related to the bonds that individuals form with the people and institutions in their lives. It is insufficient to just form ties—young people need to be active agents in these relationships. Character encompasses many assets and is related to how an individual chooses to act within the world. A well-developed character would include understanding and choosing to follow societal standards for behaviour, morals, and integrity. The fifth C is Caring, which encompasses having a sense of both sympathy and empathy for others [18].

Over time, Lerner and Lerner provided robust empirical support for this model in the 4-H Study of Positive Youth Development [4]. 4-H programs are community- and school-based youth development programs designed to build leadership and life skills through applied or "hands-on" learning opportunities for youth between 8 and 18 years of age. The name, 4-H, refers to the organization's original symbol of a four-leaf clover with an "H" on each leaf, signifying head, heart, hands, and health. Initially designed to support youth in rural and agricultural areas, 4-H now serves youth in urban, suburban, and rural communities. 4-H programs aim to create safe environments for youth to build leadership skills and personal empowerment in the following areas: Science, Technology Engineering and Math (STEM); healthy living, including physical, mental and emotional health; and active engagement in the community [22]. In 2002 and 2003, over 7000 youth in the fifth grade participated in the 4-H study from 42 states, and, to date, it has followed youth through 11th grade. This study provides empirical support for the 5Cs model, and refined the PYD measure, which assessed the five components of PYD and its relationship to youth outcomes over time, such as higher contribution to society and reductions in risk behaviour [23, 24].

The 5Cs model postulates that greater PYD assets predict positive outcomes and reduced risk behaviours [15, 18, 25]. Figure 2.1 presents the Lerner and Lerner model of PYD which focuses on the bidirectional relationship between youth and the social ecology [24, 26]. As the figure illustrates, there are internal strengths of adolescents, such as hope, connection to school, and intentional self-regulation that can promote the development of PYD assets and are related to the ability of youth to take advantage of ecological resources. Ecological assets can promote the development of PYD through supporting the development of adolescents' strengths. One

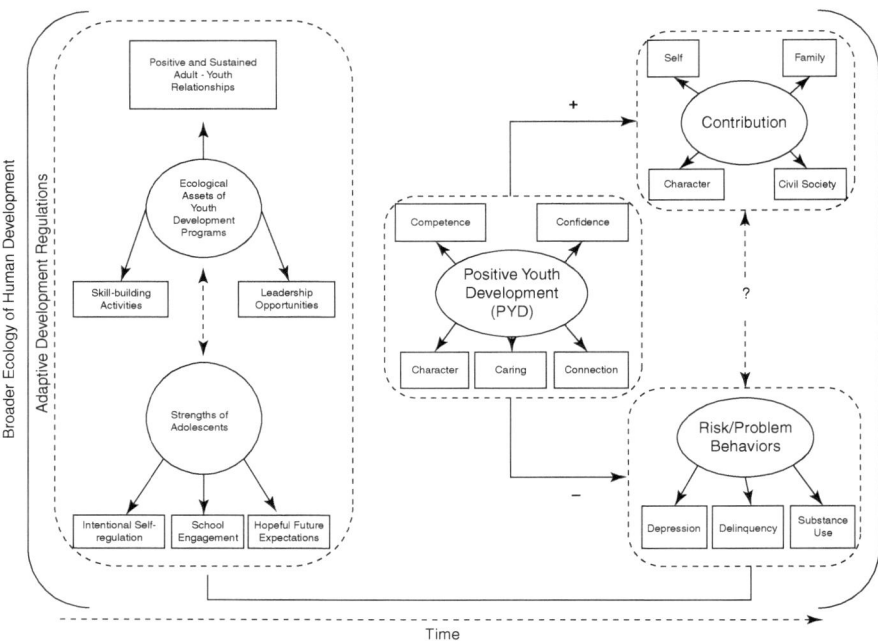

Fig. 2.1 Lerner and Lerner developmental systems model of positive youth development. (Used with permission from Richard M. Lerner; complete reference to the previous publication)

primary positive outcome is the sixth C—Contribution, defined as youth's ability to contribute to society. Youth that demonstrate high scores across the 5Cs are more likely to demonstrate greater educational and career achievement, and lower risk and problematic behaviours [24]. As a result of increases in positive internal and external attributes, the theory also postulates that youth are able to actively contribute to their own development while also enhancing their environment [27].

Empirical findings spanning a range of individual and ecological assets, including studies of mentoring, parent closeness, school connectedness and participation in spiritual or religious activities and programs have supported the PYD framework [28–31]. For example, parent-family connectedness and school connectedness are protective against risk behaviours in many domains, including substance abuse, emotional distress and violence [27]; family closeness has been associated with greater self-esteem and social competence, and fewer problem behaviours [32]; and the presence of a mentoring relationship has been shown to promote high school graduation, college attendance and employment for youth [33–35]. Other studies have focused on the quality of PYD programming provided and its impact on youth outcomes. A 2018 review of program evaluations found that programs that promoted more skill-building were associated with greater change in social conscience and character, and promoting positive social norms within the program was associated with a greater impact on youth's values, decision-making and critical thinking skills [36].

2.3   Applied Positive Youth Development and Outcomes

Similar to the paradigm shift in the understanding of health as more than the absence of illness, the National Research Council and Institute of Medicine's Committee on Community-Level Programs for Youth identified that "problem-free is not fully prepared" [15]. Meaning that youth who have multiple positive developmental assets and are not considered at-risk may not be fully prepared to take on the responsibilities of adulthood. It also means that removing a problem, such as a high-risk behaviour, may not be enough to create lasting success. Even with multiple positive factors in a young person's life, they must have opportunities to be exposed to and master a variety of life skills. This recognition encouraged programs to not only work towards the prevention of problems, but also encourage development and acquisition of life skills.

Historically, many community-based youth programs in the United States were designed to be appealing to youth of European descent [6]. Over time, the need for programs to support youth from low socioeconomic and ethnically diverse backgrounds was identified [37]. Many organizations developed new program opportunities for minority youth. Unfortunately, low-income African American, Latino, and Native American youth have not participated in youth programs to the same degree as their middle-class, European American peers [6]. While many youth programs began with a goal of reaching marginalized youth, the popularity and growth of programs for middle-class youth may have left out many marginalized youths for whom the programs were originally targeted.

As the PYD theory developed, there has been greater effort placed on determining what characterizes a PYD program. Broadly, a PYD program is one that contributes to adolescents becoming happy, healthy, and productive adults. As described in the previous section, there are multiple youth development theories with significant overlap. There is also considerable debate about *how* programs contribute to healthy adolescent development.

Empirical research supports the role of community-based youth programs in promoting positive outcomes and reducing risk behaviours for youth. The National Research Council and the Institute of Medicine also examined data regarding community programs designed to promote youth development. The findings from this report included a broad description of features of positive developmental settings including safety, appropriate structure, supportive relationships, opportunities to belong, positive social norms, support for efficacy and mattering, opportunities for skill-building, and integration of family, school, and community efforts [15]. This report built on earlier work of the Positive Youth Development Project in 1999, which examined the effectiveness of youth programs [38]. They identified a wide range of shared components including strengthening competency, building self-efficacy, and increasing healthy bonding between adults and peers. Effective programs provided structure and demonstrated consistent program delivery over the course of 9 months or more.

Roth and Brooks-Gunn built on this earlier work, examining community-based programs with the intent of describing the essential components of youth development programs [21, 26] including (1) active participant involvement; (2) a safe, caring environment that treated adolescents as responsible individuals; and (3) goals focused on developing prosocial behaviours and life skills [21]. Even when programs involve preventing problem behaviours, PYD programs have a primary goal to promote positive development. PYD programs utilize an "atmosphere of hope" ([18], p. 97) that is youth-centred and gives participants the opportunity to take on responsibility, make choices, and grow. The activities in PYD programs can provide both formal and informal opportunities for skill-building, engagement in real-life challenges, and exposure to new ideas and experiences [21]. While programs have similarities within these three characteristics, how individual organizations implement them vary.

Roth and Brooks-Gunn [21] surveyed 71 youth organizations which used PYD to further define essential programmatic components. In the program goals section, the majority of the programs had missions related to youth developing skills, connections, and competencies, while also preventing health-compromising behaviours. In the program atmosphere section, important themes included relationship-building activities to promote a supportive environment, leadership and youth decision-making to empower participants, and expectations for positive behaviour. Interestingly, programs that had a prevention goal tended to meet for fewer hours overall, were less likely to offer mentoring, and were less likely to create an empowering environment. Programs that focused on social connection demonstrated greater staff/volunteer retention. More than 75% of organizations provided programming with recreational activities, opportunities to broaden their horizon, real-life based "authentic" activities, and/or life skill, social skill or leadership training. The specific focus of the activity was less important than the opportunity to participate. Once again, programs with prevention goals tended to have lower levels of skill-building components, chances to broaden horizons, or authentic opportunities. This study also indicated that larger programs may have more difficulty in creating supportive program environments, although the budget per participant did not lead to specific program differences. Both large and small programs were able to create supportive environments that led to positive developmental opportunities.

PYD program characteristics identified by Catalano et al. [39] and Roth and Brooks-Gunn [21] overlap with Lerner's "Big Three" characteristics, which include: (1) opportunities for youth participation in and leadership of activities; (2) emphasis on the development of life skills; and (3) sustained and caring youth–adult relationships [10]. A review examining the effectiveness of programs oriented to promoting PYD among youth found that programs that demonstrated improvements in youth outcomes, such as quality of peer and adult relationships, problem solving, self-control, and academic achievement [38]. Individual features of the programs focused on strengthening social, emotional and behavioural competencies; enhancing self-efficacy; providing clear behavioural standards; increasing bonds between youth and caring adults and peers; providing opportunities for recognition and delivering programming with consistency and structure over a sustained period of time of 9 months or longer. These program features allowed AYA to gain developmental assets that led to the overall outcomes [39]. Roth and Brooks-Gunn characterize PYD programs as those that create safe, supportive, and empowering spaces that focus on skill-building, developing self-confidence and confidence for the future, and building connections with others. Similarly, Lerner's "Big Three" model provides essential components to distinguish *how* PYD programming can promote and enhance the 5Cs. While different programs may implement the "Big Three" in a variety of ways, they are important to the development of the 5Cs. Developing the 5Cs helps lead to the sixth C, Contribution, and studies have shown that the more developmental assets an individual has attained, the greater the effect on positive outcomes [40, 41].

The relationship between these characteristics and enhanced PYD continues to be an active area of research. Ramey and Rose-Krasnor [42] argued that it is important to not only examine whether or not youth participate in quality programs, but specifically how youth interact within the context of the program. They argued that it is necessary to examine in detail the interactions between youth and a program to understand the relationship between program activities and the subsequent development of PYD assets.

Policy makers and public health officials are interested in using youth development programs to reduce problem behaviours. A 2003 report by the Forum for Youth Investment focused on the importance of thinking broadly about youth development for all youth to reduce problem behaviours, promote positive outcomes, and broadly prepare youth for adulthood [43]. The importance of youth participation in programming outside of school has been incorporated into the Healthy People 2020 objectives, with the goal of increasing the proportion of youth who participate in outside of school activities by 10% [44]. Youth programs are an important tool to promote the development of youth at the local and national level.

With the growth of PYD programs, the need for evaluation has also been highlighted. A confounding factor in determining the efficacy of these programs is that, as described above, there is no set definition of a PYD program. While there are principles that have been deemed important, there are variations in the terms used to describe these principles. Additionally, simply stating that a program is PYD focused does not necessarily mean that it contains the Big Three or emphasizes growth through the 5Cs.

Given promising findings in at-risk youth, the PYD approach can be applied to other populations, such as AYA with COCC. Focusing on developing internal youth assets by building skills and competency through the experience of safe connections with caring adults, PYD programs and approaches can be applied to a variety of communities and organizations that aim to support adolescents as they transition into adulthood. In particular, this approach is especially relevant for programs or entities that serve youth with chronic conditions who would benefit from opportunities to build life skills, leadership and connections within their community.

2.4   Positive Youth Development and Chronic Conditions

More than 15% of adolescents live with childhood onset chronic conditions (COCC) including diabetes, sickle cell disease, inflammatory bowel disease, physical disabilities and other conditions [45, 46]. Along with environmental, health behavioural, and genetic changes, advances in medical technology over the past four decades have led to substantially increased life expectancy for many youth with COCC, with significantly more youth with chronic conditions now surviving into adulthood [47, 48]. With this transition to adulthood, youth with COCC face multiple challenges, including suboptimal educational, vocational and financial attainment, poor health outcomes due to inadequate self-care, halted health care transition, risk-taking behaviours, as well lower levels of psychosocial adjustment and quality of life [3, 49, 50]. Therefore, it is imperative to conceptualize ways to support this population in becoming successful young adults in all areas of life. There are many aspects of PYD that make it an ideal framework to use in programming for youth with COCC, such as focusing on youths' strengths, aligning youths' strengths with their contexts, honing skills, and promoting attributes such as competence, self-determination and self-efficacy, which have been shown to promote the successful transition to adulthood [18, 51].

A comparison of positive youth development for adolescents with and without COCC provides initial evidence that approaches used to promote positive outcomes among youth without COCC can be applied to youth with COCC. Surprisingly, there were no significant differences between adolescents with and without COCC on overall PYD or any of the 5C domains. Confirmatory factor analysis demonstrated that the same structure of PYD as measured by Lerner in the general population can be applied to youth with COCC [52]. These findings suggest that PYD-based interventions for youth without COCC are applicable to youth with COCC. An unpublished manuscript evaluating rates of participation in general youth programming among youth with and without COCC found that adolescents with COCC were just as likely as their peers without COCC to be engaged in youth programming, indicating that these programs may be sites to target PYD-based practices [53]. Another finding from the analysis indicated that Latino and other ethnic and racial minority youth were significantly less likely to participate in youth programming. Therefore, programs that serve youth with chronic conditions should take additional steps to include youth of diverse ethnic and racial backgrounds.

Historically, studies of youth with COCC have taken a problem-focused approach rather than concentrating on youths' strengths. Living with a chronic condition is often considered a challenge that one must overcome. Youth with COCC are a vulnerable population at risk of becoming over-medicalized and are especially in need of a strengths-based framework for positive growth.

Like populations for which PYD was originally conceptualized, youth with COCC are an underserved, at-risk group. Indeed, rates of delinquent behaviour are comparatively high in this population given the increased health vulnerability of these youth, and these maladaptive behaviours may have more detrimental effects [54, 55]. For example, a teenager with diabetes who uses alcohol may not recognize a low blood sugar and become comatose; a young adult with asthma who is non-adherent with their treatment regimen is at risk of death from a fatal asthma attack. For youth with COCC, the stakes are higher in the case of risky behaviours, and therefore the need for targeted intervention is even more imperative. The PYD approach has been used to promote positive health behaviours and decrease risk behaviours for at-risk youth in the areas of sexual health and substance use [56, 57]. Analysis of these programs indicates that wellbeing in adolescence is associated with decreased health risk and improved general health in young adulthood for youth without COCC [58]. Based on this data, youth with COCC could substantially benefit from PYD-based programs in terms of health outcomes in the context of risky behaviours.

The PYD framework of aligning youths' strengths with resources in their environment to promote optimal development has been applied to high-risk populations of youth with success in promoting positive outcomes. For youth with COCC, leveraging ecological assets is even more essential. Youth with COCC are often isolated from their community [59] related to a number of factors including school absences [53], lack of programs that can accommodate youth with disabilities, higher rates of mental illness, or other challenges [60]. The PYD approach enhances the alignment between an individual's strengths and environmental resources, thus fostering community, which is critical for youth with COCC. It has been shown that enhancing community connectedness, especially in schools, promotes educational attainment for youth with COCC [34], a critical factor in future financial stability and success in adulthood. Similarly, evaluations of PYD programs have demonstrated improved mental and physical health, enhanced resilience, and overall quality of life for youth without COCC [38, 61]. While some studies have shown higher quality of life among adults with serious health conditions, known as the disability paradox [62], research has also found higher rates of mental health conditions among youth with COCC compared to youth without COCC [60, 63]; therefore, the benefits of PYD programming have the potential to be extended to the chronic illness population with valuable implications.

For positive development to occur, youth must become activated, motivated and engaged in their own development [17]. According to Larson, PYD assumes that a young person has the inherent capacity to derive motivation through challenge, which serves to galvanize that individual's active engagement in their development. Many youths with COCC face challenges on a daily basis related to their condition, which may provide the motivation to catalyze engagement. For youth with COCC, this is especially important given the additional burden of caring for their chronic condition and its implications on health outcomes. If youth are motivated to engage in their development, that motivation may extend to increased engagement in their health management and health promotion leading to improved overall wellbeing.

AYA with COCC struggle with the transition to adulthood in vocational, educational and financial areas. They are less likely to graduate from college, obtain gainful employment, and earn less income compared to their healthy peers [64, 2, 3]. In addition, the period of healthcare transition from paediatric to adult medicine presents a high-risk period for youth with COCC and is associated with increases in morbidity and mortality [65–67].

Transition readiness, or the ability of adolescents and their family to engage in the process of moving from paediatric to adult care, has been conceptualized as a developmental skill important to consider in the context of other developmental tasks that adolescents with chronic conditions are acquiring as they mature [68]. Transition readiness has been linked to other youth development constructs that are associated with PYD including intentional self-regulation (ISR) and hopeful future expectations (HFE). ISR involves the process of selecting and setting goals, using skills to optimize one's chances of successfully achieving those goals, and compensating or altering one's trajectory if attempts at actualizing goals fail [69]. ISR is a modifiable developmental skill that could be promoted with PYD-oriented programming and is particularly relevant to youth with COCC who may have to adjust life goals in the face of condition-related challenges. ISR has been shown to be associated with transition readiness in youth with COCC [68]. Self-regulation has been conceptualized as instrumental to chronic condition self-management via its effect on individual and interpersonal processes [70]. HFE may facilitate the development of transition readiness as well given its influential effect on ISR [71]. Since more advanced developmental skills are tied to enhanced transition readiness, encouraging positive youth development for youth with COCC may also enhance transition outcomes, both related to healthcare transition and transition into adulthood.

According to the PYD framework, successful youth outcomes include the development of attributes of competence, confidence, character, social connectedness and compassion, known as the 5Cs described above [39]. Competence and confidence are two internal PYD assets that are important for promoting and ensuring optimal self-management through activation—a critical skill for youth with COCC. Patient activation is defined as the individual's knowledge, skill and confidence in management of their own health [72], and there is increasing evidence supporting the importance of activation in promoting positive outcomes for people with chronic conditions [73, 74]. Healthcare transition is defined as a "multifaceted, active process that attends to the medical, psychosocial, and educational or vocational needs of adolescents as they move from the child-focused to the adult-focused health-care system"; it involves the development of autonomy and independence, as well as transition in other areas of the youth's life, such as school, work, and the community [75]. Higher activation scores on the Patient Activation Measure have predicted transition readiness in a study of AYA with rheumatic disease [76] suggesting that targeting activation could improve healthcare transition. Health literacy and numeracy scores in this same cohort did not predict transition readiness, consistent with the finding that knowledge alone is not sufficient to promote improved patient engagement and outcomes [77]. For youth with COCC, it is not only paramount that they understand their condition, symptoms, and management, but that they have the confidence to carry out their treatment plans and advocate for themselves in order to become successful and healthy adults. Both competence and confidence have been associated with enhanced patient activation [72] and are promoted through PYD programming.

Hibbard et al. [72] conceptualized a 4-stage developmental model of activation: (1) believing in the importance of the individual's role in their healthcare, (2) having the *confidence* and *knowledge* (or competence) necessary to take action, (3) taking action to maintain and improve one's health, and (4) staying the course under stress. Of note, "staying the course under stress" can be understood as ISR in the PYD framework. Higher levels of patient activation have been associated with decreased unnecessary healthcare utilization and improved health outcomes [73]. It is clear that essential components of PYD influence activation. Thus, improving positive development in youth with COCC on a broad level may improve transition readiness and health outcomes via patient activation [68].

PYD programming for youth with COCC fosters the development of successful young adults who are active contributors to their communities, and is an opportune forum for helping youth become active and engaged self-managers of their condition and their lives. The effectiveness of the PYD approach in fostering positive outcomes for youth with COCC was examined by Maslow and Chung [78] in a systematic review of programs for youth with COCC that employed principles of PYD. Fourteen youth programs (15 studies) were identified that included at least one core component of PYD. Only three studies were considered comprehensive (included all three core elements of PYD programs: opportunities for leadership, skill-building and sustained relationships with adult mentors). Four programs were mentoring-based (promoted sustained youth–adult relationships), and seven focused on youth leadership (youth were actively involved in program leadership). Below, we present different types of programs that could be leveraged to support PYD in youth with COCC based on this review of the literature [78]. The review identified programs employing some combination of PYD principles and underscores the variety of programs that could be harnessed to promote PYD.

2.4.1 Mentorship

By harnessing the connections among AYA, peer-based mentorship provides a mechanism to promote PYD. We recommend intervention models that integrate young adults who have successfully navigated the transition to adult care to serve in leadership roles to support their peers in navigating this arduous transition process to adult healthcare and adulthood. This model could be supported by one-to-one mentoring models in which mentors are individually matched with AYA, or in group settings with multiple mentors and youth meeting together. Peer-based mentoring interventions have shown to promote positive outcomes for AYA with chronic conditions, such as improved self-efficacy, empowerment and wellbeing [79], as well as improved self-care advocacy and reduced loneliness [80].

Group-based mentorship has been shown to promote PYD. For example, The Adolescent Leadership Council (TALC) and Adolescents Transitioning to Leadership and Success (ATLAS) programs, which are healthcare transition focused leadership programs based in hospital settings, bring together college mentors and high school participants for monthly meetings. The programs encompass the "Big Three" PYD components and provide the opportunity for college mentors and participants to discuss ways to adaptively grow up with a chronic condition. Topic areas are chosen by youth participants; examples include 'talking to friends about one's chronic condition', 'speaking with the doctor independently', and 'identifying and obtaining accommodations in school'. College-aged mentors help develop programming activities, such as role plays, ice breakers, and instructional games. These programs also include a skill-building component, which allows participants to gain confidence and competence in skills that are related to successfully transitioning into adulthood and the adult healthcare system. With the oversight of medical staff, college age-mentors are able to provide support to high school participants. Mentors share their own experiences to help guide and support high school participants. These programs have been associated with positive outcomes and promote PYD [80, 81].

The Chronic Illness Peers Support Program (ChIPS), a well-established program located in Australia, also includes the three core components of a PYD program [82]. Following participation in weekly group sessions, youth can choose to participate in various social, educational, and leadership-based activities throughout the year. This program provides opportunities for youth to take on multiple leadership roles, such as serving as a group mentor/co-facilitator, fundraising, and engaging in advocacy. With activities occurring year-round, youth can develop sustained relationships with adults throughout the year, and develop a variety of important skills.

2.4.2   Leadership

Traditional leadership-based programs provide another mechanism to promote PYD elements. The leadership programs included in the systematic review described above include Outward Bound, camp- and school-based programs, which provide youth with COCC an opportunity to serve as leaders, support one another, and participate in program development.

Outward bound programs provide youth the opportunity to learn and develop while engaging in outdoor activities. Programs for youth with chronic illness have been effective in promoting short-term and long-term outcomes, including improvements in leadership, self-concept, and school attendance. The British Outward Bound program, for instance, was developed for youth with type 1 diabetes, in which youth participate in outdoor excursions while also having to manage their diabetes care [83]. This provides the opportunity for youth to learn essential self-management and problem-solving skills in a variety of conditions [78, 83]. It also provides an opportunity for youth to serve as leaders and support one another during challenging outdoor activities.

Another context in which to promote PYD is the summer camp setting. Summer camps dedicated to youth with COCC serve a large portion of youth with COCC [84]. Youth who attend camp are already engaged and have established relationships with camp counsellors and staff. Camps designed for youth with COCC could leverage these relationships to develop a PYD-based program by complementing youth–adult sustained relationships with skill-building and leadership opportunities [84]. A recent systematic review evaluated all research studies conducted of camps for youth with COCC over the past century in the United States and examined whether the camps utilize PYD-based principles. Of the 425 studies reviewed, over 50% contained all three principles of PYD, and over 90% included at least two of the three components. Although studies did not directly address the three principles, this helps to underscore the opportunity for camps to integrate PYD programming [84]. Beyond the campers, research suggests that AYA counsellors with chronic conditions may also benefit from camp in terms of their condition self-management. At a camp for youth with diabetes, AYA counsellors with diabetes were found to have significant reductions in Haemoglobin A1C, a marker of blood sugar control, over 6–10 weeks at camp [85].

Maslow and Chung [78] highlight the need for more rigorous research to evaluate the impact of programs on the promotion of medical, healthcare transition, and psychosocial outcomes for youth with COCC. While all studies in the review assessed psychosocial outcomes, only four respective studies examined medical outcomes (e.g. glycaemic control, weight loss) and healthcare transition outcomes (e.g. self-advocacy, self-management). Psychosocial adjustment and empowerment improved in a mentoring program for youth with disabilities. Other studies demonstrated no change in self-worth, coping, self-esteem, locus of control and diabetes adjustment. These findings underline the lack of rigorous PYD-based program evaluations in AYAs with COCC, which limits the ability to comprehensively evaluate the efficacy of PYD-based programs.

2.5 Key Recommendations for Practice

Based on the current literature and our team's 20+ years of PYD programming for AYA with COCC, our recommendations are both broad and specific. Just as PYD has been conceptualized in many ways, with a variety of components, implementing PYD in practice can be achieved in myriad forms. In order to determine how to best utilize PYD, it is important to understand both the setting and overall goals. While most of the PYD research has been on structured programs, the same principles may be applicable in other settings.

When developing interventions for AYA with COCC, we recommend integrating the Big Three components of PYD principles. Firstly, this includes providing opportunities for AYA participants to establish positive and stable long-term relationships with adult role models. Secondly, integrating skill-building components into programing is essential; these could include skills specific to living with a chronic illness, such as self-management (i.e. treatment regimen adherence) and healthcare navigation (i.e. self-advocacy in the physician's office), as well as skills related to AYA more generally, such as educational and vocational related abilities. Third, programming should be intentional about providing leadership opportunities for AYA. There are various ways to provide leadership opportunities such as involving

AYA in program planning, incorporating AYA in mentorship roles, and enabling youth to develop and lead programs.

There is not one specific way to incorporate all three PYD principles into a program. We encourage program developers to be creative and innovative in forming developmentally appropriate, PYD-based programs. For many programs serving AYA with chronic conditions, modifications to current programming may lead to incorporation of more PYD components. Programs can complete self-assessments on how well they incorporate the Big Three into their current offerings, and then integrate additional principle(s) into the intervention model. For example, an Outward Bound program for AYA with chronic conditions may already be integrating sustained adult-youth relationships and skill building, and may consider incorporating leadership opportunities, such as enabling AYA to plan excursion or serve as mentors. PYD-based programs for youth with COCC have been implemented by individuals with various levels of expertise in a range of settings including the hospital, school, community, and online.

The Big Three are associated with promoting internal attributes consistent with Lerner's 5Cs: competence, character, confidence, connection, and compassion. Developmental theory and research have shown that as AYA develop more assets, their outcomes improve. Promoting the 5Cs may identify youth strengths and enhance assets, which can help AYA with COCC to thrive. ISR and HFE are two components described above that have been linked to PYD and enhanced transition readiness, and may be related to improved health outcomes. If it is not possible to integrate the Big Three into interventions, identifying which components of the 5Cs, ISR, and HFE best fit within the goals of an organization or program will allow for more targeted interventions. Additionally, being aware of the diversity of the target group will be necessary in order to create culturally appropriate and successful programs.

While current studies examining PYD programs for youth with COCC have many shortcomings, such as lack of control groups, small sample sizes, and limited follow-up, this creates an opportunity for growth. Moving forward, it is critical for researchers to use rigorous methods across studies and sites to better capture the development of positive youth attributes in AYA with chronic conditions over time. Rigorous methodologies aside from the standard randomized control trials may be more realistic, especially as many organizations that provide programming do not participate in research. Identifying new models to study these varied programs may help to mitigate these concerns while also serving as many AYA with COCC as possible. While there are currently a few measures to evaluate PYD that can be utilized for both informal assessment and research, further validation and study is needed.

We also recommend integrating aspects of PYD into healthcare practice. While healthcare providers are not necessarily mentors, they are adults in a young person's life who often have a positive influence longitudinally. Encouraging AYA with COCC to have a larger role in their healthcare may improve their motivation and compliance. Incorporating skill-building opportunities into office visits, such as answering health questions, giving a medical history, and/or making an appointment independently in the absence of parents, may help empower AYA with COCC and enhance both confidence and competence. When possible, including AYA with COCC in decision-making, both for their own care and for broader clinic or systems issues may help promote leadership. These changes to practice may help AYA with COCC to develop more assets, which in turn may improve health outcomes.

2.6   Conclusion

Due to great medical advancement, the majority of youth diagnosed with a chronic condition will now survive into adulthood. These medical achievements have led to a greater focus on the long-term outcomes in this population. Developmentally based theories have been critical in moving from mitigating current physical and psychological symptomatology to promoting optimal development. PYD is one theory that can help to inform how to best support adaptive long-term development for youth with COCC. This chapter provides a historical overview of PYD, as well as its theoretical underpinnings. Lerner and Lerner's 5Cs model is introduced as an empirically supported approach, which posits that individual youth assets can predict long-term outcomes in at-risk youth. Initial evidence is described that demonstrates a good fit for applying Lerner and Lerner's 5Cs framework to youth with chronic conditions.

In sum, PYD can be leveraged to achieve optimal development of AYA with COCC and presents an area ripe for investigation in this population. This chapter presents the current state of knowledge on PYD programs in AYA with COCC. The recommendations for practice are outlined to provide guidance for professionals working with this population in various settings to promote PYD. While clinical implications for the importance of PYD in this population are highlighted, research in this area remains limited. This chapter should serve as a foundation for future research to better understand and promote PYD in AYA with COCC.

References

1. American Academy of Pediatrics, American Academy of Family Physicians, & American College of Physicians-American Society of Internal Medicine. A consensus statement on health care transitions for young adults with special health care needs. Pediatrics. 2002;110(6 Pt 2):1304–6.
2. Gledhill J, Rangel L, Garralda E. Surviving chronic physical illness: psychosocial outcome in adult life. Arch Dis Child. 2000;83(2):104–10. https://doi.org/10.1136/adc.83.2.104.
3. Maslow GR, Haydon A, McRee AL, Ford CA, Halpern CT. Growing up with a chronic illness: social success, educational/vocational distress. J Adolesc Health. 2011;49(2):206–12. https://doi.org/10.1016/j.jadohealth.2010.12.001.
4. Lerner RM, Lerner JV. The positive development of youth: report of the findings from the first eight years of the 4-H study of positive youth development. Chevy Chase, MD: Tufts University. Institute for Applied Research in Youth Development; National 4-H Council (U.S.); 2012. https://www.researchconnections.org/childcare/resources/24310.
5. Samuel HD. Troubled passage: the labor movement and the Fair Labor Standards Act. Mon Labor Rev. 2000;123(12):32.
6. Russell ST, Campen KV. Diversity and inclusion in youth development: what we can learn from marginalized young people. J Youth Dev. 2011;6(3):94–106. https://doi.org/10.5195/jyd.2011.177.

7. The Fair Labor Standards Act of 1938, no. 75–718, Washington, DC: U.S. Dept. of Labor, Wage and Hour Division; n.d.
8. Walker JA, Alberti Gambone M, Walker KC. Reflections of a century of youth development research and practice. J Youth Dev. 2011;6:11. https://doi.org/10.5195/jyd.2011.172.
9. Damon W. What is positive youth development? Ann Am Acad Pol Soc Sci. 2004;591(1):13–24. https://doi.org/10.1177/0002716203260092.
10. Lerner RM. Liberty: thriving and civic engagement among America's youth. Philadelphia, PA: SAGE Publications Inc.; 2004. https://doi.org/10.4135/9781452233581. ISBN: 9780761929840.
11. Lerner RM, Abo-Zena MM, Bebiroglu N, Brittian A, Lynch AD, Issac SS. Positive youth development: contemporary theoretical perspectives. In: DiClemente RJ, Santelli JS, Crosby RA, editors. Adolescent health: understanding and preventing risk behaviors. 1st ed. San Francisco, CA: Jossey-Bass; 2009. p. 115–28. https://ebookcentral.proquest.com/lib/duke/detail.action?docID=433714.
12. Lerner RM, Almerigi JB, Theokas C, Lerner JV. Positive youth development a view of the issues. J Early Adolesc. 2005a;25(1):10–6. https://doi.org/10.1177/0272431604273211.
13. Damon W, Menon J, Cotton Bronk K. The development of purpose during adolescence. Appl Dev Sci. 2003;7(3):119–28. https://doi.org/10.1207/S1532480XADS0703_2.
14. Benson PL, Scales PC, Syvertsen AK. Chapter 8—The contribution of the developmental assets framework to positive youth development theory and practice. In: Lerner RM, Lerner JV, Benson JB, editors. Advances in child development and behavior, vol. 41. Amsterdam: Elsevier; 2011. p. 197–230. https://doi.org/10.1016/B978-0-12-386492-5.00008-7.
15. Eccles J, Gootman JA, editors. Community programs to promote youth development. Washington, DC: National Academy Press; 2002. https://find.library.duke.edu/catalog/DUKE003068237.
16. Piaget J. Biology and knowledge. Chicago, IL: University of Chicago Press; 1967.
17. Larson R. Positive youth development, willful adolescents, and mentoring. J Community Psychol. 2006;34(6):677–89. https://doi.org/10.1002/jcop.20123.
18. Lerner RM. The positive youth development perspective: theoretical and empirical bases of a strengths-based approach to adolescent development. The Oxford handbook of positive psychology. Oxford: Oxford University Press; 2009. https://doi.org/10.1093/oxfordhb/9780195187243.013.0014.
19. Lerner RM, Fisher CB, Weinberg RA. Toward a science for and of the people: promoting civil society through the application of developmental science. Child Dev. 2000;71(1):11–20. https://doi.org/10.1111/1467-8624.00113.
20. Pittman K, Irby M, Ferber T. Unfinished business: further reflections on a decade of promoting youth development. In: Benson PL, Pittman KJ, editors. Trends in youth development: visions, realities and challenges. New York, NY: Springer; 2001. p. 3–50.
21. Roth JL, Brooks-Gunn J. Youth development programs: risk, prevention and policy. J Adolesc Health. 2003;32(3):170–82. https://doi.org/10.1016/s1054-139x(02)00421-4.
22. 4-H Youth Programs—STEM, Health, Agriculture & Civic Engagement. 4-H. n.d.. https://4-h.org/parents/programs-at-a-glance/.
23. Bowers EP, Li Y, Kiely MK, Brittian A, Lerner JV, Lerner RM. The five Cs model of positive youth development: a longitudinal analysis of confirmatory factor structure and measurement invariance. J Youth Adolesc. 2010;39(7):720–35. https://doi.org/10.1007/s10964-010-9530-9.
24. Lerner RM, von Eye A, Lerner JV, Lewin-Bizan S, Bowers EP. Special issue introduction: the meaning and measurement of thriving: a view of the issues. J Youth Adolesc. 2010;39(7):707–19. https://doi.org/10.1007/s10964-010-9531-8.
25. Bowers EP, Geldhof GJ. Promoting positive youth development: lessons from the 4-H study. Cham: Springer Verlag; 2015. https://find.library.duke.edu/catalog/DUKE006643418.
26. Lerner RM, Lerner JV, Lewin-Bizan S, Bowers EP, Boyd MJ, Mueller MK, Schmid KL, Napolitano CM. Positive youth development: processes, programs, and problematics. J Youth Dev. 2011;6(3):38–62. https://doi.org/10.5195/jyd.2011.174.

27. Resnick MD, Bearman PS, Blum RW, Bauman KE, Harris KM, Jones J, Tabor J, Beuhring T, Sieving RE, Shew M, Ireland M, Bearinger LH, Udry JR. Protecting adolescents from harm: findings from the national longitudinal study on adolescent health. JAMA. 1997;278(10):823–32. https://doi.org/10.1001/jama.1997.03550100049038.
28. Bond L, Butler H, Thomas L, Carlin J, Glover S, Bowes G, Patton G. Social and school connectedness in early secondary school as predictors of late teenage substance use, mental health, and academic outcomes. J Adolesc Health. 2007;40(4):357.e9–357.e18. https://doi.org/10.1016/j.jadohealth.2006.10.013.
29. Nonnemaker JM, McNeely CA, Blum RW. Public and private domains of religiosity and adolescent health risk behaviors: evidence from the National Longitudinal Study of Adolescent Health. Soc Sci Med. 2003;57(11):2049–54. https://doi.org/10.1016/S0277-9536(03)00096-0.
30. Pittman LD, Richmond A. Academic and psychological functioning in late adolescence: the importance of school belonging. J Exp Educ. 2007;75(4):270–90. https://doi.org/10.3200/JEXE.75.4.270-292.
31. Saewyc EM, Homma Y, Skay CL, Bearinger LH, Resnick MD, Reis E. Protective factors in the lives of bisexual adolescents in North America. Am J Public Health. 2009;99(1):110–7. https://doi.org/10.2105/AJPH.2007.123109.
32. Youngblade LM, Theokas C, Schulenberg J, Curry L, Huang IC, Novak M. Risk and promotive factors in families, schools, and communities: a contextual model of positive youth development in adolescence. Pediatrics. 2007;119(Suppl 1):S47–53. https://doi.org/10.1542/peds.2006-2089H.
33. Erickson LD, McDonald S, Elder GH. Informal mentors and education: complementary or compensatory resources? Sociol Educ. 2009;82(4):344–67. https://doi.org/10.1177/003804070908200403.
34. Maslow G, Haydon AA, McRee AL, Halpern CT. Protective connections and educational attainment among young adults with childhood-onset chronic illness*. J Sch Health. 2012;82(8):364–70. https://doi.org/10.1111/j.1746-1561.2012.00710.x.
35. McDonald S, Erickson LD, Johnson MK, Elder GH. Informal mentoring and young adult employment. Soc Sci Res. 2007;36(4):1328–47. https://doi.org/10.1016/j.ssresearch.2007.01.008.
36. Smischney TM, Roberts MA, Gliske K, Borden LM, Perkins DF. Developing youth competencies: the impact of program quality. J Youth Dev. 2018;13(4):29. https://doi.org/10.5195/jyd.2018.587.
37. Scholl J, Paster A. Locating, analyzing and making available a century of 4-H research studies, 1911-2011. J Youth Dev. 2011;6(3):63–79. https://doi.org/10.5195/jyd.2011.175.
38. Catalano RF, Berglund ML, Ryan JAM, Lonczak HS, Hawkins JD. Positive youth development in the United States: research findings on evaluations of positive youth development programs. Ann Am Acad Pol Soc Sci. 2004;591(1):98–124. https://doi.org/10.1177/0002716203260102.
39. Catalano RF, Berglund ML, Ryan JAM, Lonczak HS, Hawkins JD. Positive youth development in the United States: research findings on evaluations of positive youth development programs. Prev Treat. 2002;5(1):15. https://doi.org/10.1037/1522-3736.5.1.515a.
40. Jelicic H, Bobek DL, Phelps E, Lerner RM, Lerner JV. Using positive youth development to predict contribution and risk behaviors in early adolescence: findings from the first two waves of the 4-H study of positive youth development. Int J Behav Dev. 2007;31(3):263–73. https://doi.org/10.1177/0165025407076439.
41. Lerner RM, Lerner JV, Almerigi JB, Theokas C, Gestsdottir S, Naudeau S, Jelicic H, Alberts A, Ma L, Smith LM, Bobek DL, Richman-Raphael D, Simpson I, Christiansen ED, Von Eye A. Positive youth development, participation in community youth development programs, and community contributions of fifth-grade adolescents: findings from the first wave of the 4-H study of positive youth development. J Early Adolesc. 2005b;25(1):17–71. https://doi.org/10.1177/0272431604272461.
42. Ramey HL, Rose-Krasnor L. Contexts of structured youth activities and positive youth development. Child Dev Perspect. 2012;6(1):85–91. https://doi.org/10.1111/j.1750-8606.2011.00219.x.

43. Johnson Pittman K, Irby M, Tolman J, Yohalem N, Ferber T. Preventing problems, promoting development, encouraging engagement: competing priorities or inseparable goals? Based upon Johnson Pittman, K. & Irby, M. (1996). Preventing problems or promoting development? Washington, DC: The Forum for Youth Investment, Impact Strategies, Inc; 2003.
44. U.S. Department of Health and Human Services. Healthy People 2020. n.d.. https://www.healthypeople.gov/.
45. Newacheck PW, Strickland B, Shonkoff JP, Perrin JM, McPherson M, McManus M, Lauver C, Fox H, Arango P. An epidemiologic profile of children with special health care needs. Pediatrics. 1998;102(1 Pt 1):117–23. https://doi.org/10.1542/peds.102.1.117.
46. van Dyck PC, Kogan MD, McPherson MG, Weissman GR, Newacheck PW. Prevalence and characteristics of children with special health care needs. JAMA Pediatr. 2004;158(9):884–90. https://doi.org/10.1001/archpedi.158.9.884.
47. Blum RW. Transition to adult health care: setting the stage. J Adolesc Health. 1995;17(1):3–5. https://doi.org/10.1016/1054-139x(95)00073-2.
48. Perrin JM, Bloom SR, Gortmaker SL. The increase of childhood chronic conditions in the united states. JAMA. 2007;297(24):2755–9. https://doi.org/10.1001/jama.297.24.2755.
49. Hazel E, Zhang X, Duffy CM, Campillo S. High rates of unsuccessful transfer to adult care among young adults with juvenile idiopathic arthritis. Pediatr Rheumatol Online J. 2010;8:2. https://doi.org/10.1186/1546-0096-8-2.
50. Hudson MM, Findlay S. Health-risk behaviors and health promotion in adolescent and young adult cancer survivors. Cancer. 2006;107(S7):1695–701. https://doi.org/10.1002/cncr.22103.
51. Ryan RM, Deci EL. Self-determination theory and the facilitation of intrinsic motivation, social development, and well-being. Am Psychol. 2000;55(1):68–78.
52. Maslow GR, Hill SN, Pollock MD. Comparison of positive youth development for youth with chronic conditions with healthy peers. J Adolesc Health. 2016;59(6):716–21. https://doi.org/10.1016/j.jadohealth.2016.08.004.
53. Sendak MD, Hill SN, Pollock MD, Brotkin SM, Maslow GR. An examination of participation in youth programs for adolescents with chronic illness. Unpublished manuscript. Durham, NC: Duke University; 2018a.
54. Hollen PJ, Hobbie WL, Donnangelo SF, Shannon S, Erickson J. Substance use risk behaviors and decision-making skills among cancer-surviving adolescents. J Pediatr Oncol Nurs. 2007;24(5):264–73. https://doi.org/10.1177/1043454207304910.
55. Valencia LS, Cromer BA. Sexual activity and other high-risk behaviors in adolescents with chronic illness: a review. J Pediatr Adolesc Gynecol. 2000;13(2):53–64. https://doi.org/10.1016/S1083-3188(00)00004-8.
56. Gavin LE, Catalano RF, David-Ferdon C, Gloppen KM, Markham CM. A review of positive youth development programs that promote adolescent sexual and reproductive health. J Adolesc Health. 2010;46(3 Suppl):S75–91. https://doi.org/10.1016/j.jadohealth.2009.11.215.
57. Guerra NG, Bradshaw CP. Linking the prevention of problem behaviors and positive youth development: core competencies for positive youth development and risk prevention. New Dir Child Adolesc Dev. 2008;2008(122):1–17. https://doi.org/10.1002/cd.225.
58. Hoyt LT, Chase-Lansdale PL, Mcdade TW, Adam EK. Positive youth, healthy adults: does positive well-being in adolescence predict better perceived health and fewer risky health behaviors in young adulthood? J Adolesc Health. 2012;50(1):66–73. https://doi.org/10.1016/j.jadohealth.2011.05.002.
59. Suris JC, Michaud PA, Viner R. The adolescent with a chronic condition. Part I: developmental issues. Arch Dis Child. 2004;89(10):938–42. https://doi.org/10.1136/adc.2003.045369.
60. Kline-Simon AH, Weisner C, Sterling S. Point prevalence of co-occurring behavioral health conditions and associated chronic disease burden among adolescents. J Am Acad Child Adolesc Psychiatry. 2016;55(5):408–14. https://doi.org/10.1016/j.jaac.2016.02.008.
61. Sanders J, Munford R, Thimasarn-Anwar T, Liebenberg L, Ungar M. The role of positive youth development practices in building resilience and enhancing wellbeing for at-risk youth. Child Abuse Negl. 2015;42:40–53. https://doi.org/10.1016/j.chiabu.2015.02.006.

62. Albrecht GL, Devlieger PJ. The disability paradox: high quality of life against all odds. Soc Sci Med. 1999;48(8):977–88. https://doi.org/10.1016/S0277-9536(98)00411-0.
63. Pinquart M, Shen Y. Depressive symptoms in children and adolescents with chronic physical illness: an updated meta-analysis. J Pediatr Psychol. 2011;36(4):375–84. https://doi.org/10.1093/jpepsy/jsq104.
64. Blum RW, Hirsh D, Kastner T, Quint RD, Sandler AD, Anderson SM, Britto M, Brunstrom J, Buchanan GA, Burke R, Chamberlain JK, Cooper B, Davidow D, Evans T, Gloss T, Hackett P, Harr P, Kiernan W, Levey E, Ziring P. A consensus statement on health care transitions for young adults with special health care needs. Pediatrics. 2002;110(6 Pt 2):1304–6.
65. Garvey KC, Wolpert HA, Rhodes ET, Laffel LM, Kleinman K, Beste MG, Wolfsdorf JI, Finkelstein JA. Health care transition in patients with type 1 diabetes: young adult experiences and relationship to glycemic control. Diabetes Care. 2012;35(8):1716–22. https://doi.org/10.2337/dc11-2434.
66. Watson AR. Non-compliance and transfer from paediatric to adult transplant unit. Pediatr Nephrol. 2000;14(6):469–72. https://doi.org/10.1007/s004670050794.
67. Wojciechowski EA, Hurtig A, Dorn L. A natural history study of adolescents and young adults with sickle cell disease as they transfer to adult care: a need for case management services. J Pediatr Nurs. 2002;17(1):18–27. https://doi.org/10.1053/jpdn.2002.30930.
68. Hart LC, Pollock M, Hill S, Maslow G. Association of transition readiness to intentional self-regulation and hopeful future expectations in youth with illness. Acad Pediatr. 2017;17(4):450–5. https://doi.org/10.1016/j.acap.2016.12.004.
69. Freund AM, Baltes PB. Life-management strategies of selection, optimization, and compensation: measurement by self-report and construct validity. J Pers Soc Psychol. 2002;82(4):642–62.
70. Lansing AH, Berg CA. Adolescent self-regulation as a foundation for chronic illness self-management. J Pediatr Psychol. 2014;39(10):1091–6. https://doi.org/10.1093/jpepsy/jsu067.
71. Schmid KL, Phelps E, Lerner RM. Constructing positive futures: modeling the relationship between adolescents' hopeful future expectations and intentional self regulation in predicting positive youth development. J Adolesc. 2011;34(6):1127–35. https://doi.org/10.1016/j.adolescence.2011.07.009.
72. Hibbard JH, Stockard J, Mahoney ER, Tusler M. Development of the patient activation measure (PAM): conceptualizing and measuring activation in patients and consumers. Health Serv Res. 2004;39(4p1):1005–26. https://doi.org/10.1111/j.1475-6773.2004.00269.x.
73. Greene J, Hibbard JH, Sacks R, Overton V, Parrotta CD. When patient activation levels change, health outcomes and costs change, too. Health Aff. 2015;34(3):431–7. https://doi.org/10.1377/hlthaff.2014.0452.
74. Shively MJ, Gardetto NJ, Kodiath MF, Kelly A, Smith TL, Stepnowsky C, Maynard C, Larson CB. Effect of patient activation on self-management in patients with heart failure. J Cardiovasc Nurs. 2013;28(1):20–34. https://doi.org/10.1097/JCN.0b013e318239f9f9.
75. Blum RW, Garell D, Hodgman CH, Jorissen TW, Okinow NA, Orr DP, Slap GB. Transition from child-centered to adult health-care systems for adolescents with chronic conditions. A position paper of the Society for Adolescent Medicine. J Adolesc Health. 1993;14(7):570–6. https://doi.org/10.1016/1054-139X(93)90143-D.
76. Lazaroff SM, Meara A, Tompkins MK, Peters E, Ardoin SP. How do health literacy, numeric competencies, and patient activation relate to transition readiness in adolescents and young adults with rheumatic diseases. Arthr Care Res. 2018;71(9):1264–9. https://doi.org/10.1002/acr.23739.
77. Hibbard J. Patient activation and health literacy: what's the difference? How do each contribute to health outcomes. Stud Health Technol Inform. 2017;240:251–62.
78. Maslow GR, Chung RJ. Systematic review of positive youth development programs for adolescents with chronic illness. Pediatrics. 2013;131(5):e1605–18. https://doi.org/10.1542/peds.2012-1615.
79. Powers LE, Turner A, Ellison R, Matuszewski J, Wilson R, Phillips A, Rein C. A multi-component intervention to promote adolescent self-determination. J Rehabil. 2001;67(4):13–9.

80. Maslow G, Adams C, Willis M, Neukirch J, Herts K, Froehlich W, Calleson D, Rickerby M. An evaluation of a positive youth development program for adolescents with chronic illness. J Adolesc Health. 2013;52(2):179–85. https://doi.org/10.1016/j.jadohealth.2012.06.020.
81. Maslow G, Hill S, Rozycki A, Sadun R, Sendowski M, Neukirch J. Character development pilot evaluation of two programs for youth with chronic illness. J Youth Dev. 2015;10(3):115–26. https://doi.org/10.5195/jyd.2015.12.
82. Olsson CA, Boyce MF, Toumbourou JW, Sawyer SM. The role of peer support in facilitating psychosocial adjustment to chronic illness in adolescence. Clin Child Psychol Psychiatry. 2005;10(1):78–87. https://doi.org/10.1177/1359104505048793.
83. Hillson RM. Diabetes outward bound mountain course, eskdale, cumbria. Diabet Med. 1984;1(1):59–63. https://doi.org/10.1111/j.1464-5491.1984.tb01925.x.
84. Sendak MD, Schilstra C, Tye E, Brotkin S, Maslow G. Positive youth development at camps for youth with chronic illness: a systematic review of the literature. J Youth Dev. 2018b;13(1–2):201–15. https://doi.org/10.5195/jyd.2018.551.
85. Manning AS, Pollock M, Clements B, Furutani E, Brotkin S, Mansfield J, Kupersmidt J, Fritz G, Maslow G. Young adult counselors with diabetes at diabetes camps: the effect of being a peer mentor on counselors' health behavior. J Youth Dev. 2018;13(1–2):250–65. https://doi.org/10.5195/jyd.2018.540.

Jane N. T. Sattoe and AnneLoes van Staa

3.1   Introduction

The developmental context of young people with chronic conditions makes their situation different from people who are being diagnosed with a chronic condition at a later age. This also reflects in their challenges for learning and practicing self-management and the support they need. In Chap. 1, the broad definition of self-management was outlined as follows: "the individual's ability to manage the symptoms, treatment, physical and psychosocial consequences and lifestyle changes inherent in living with a chronic condition" [1].

Growing up with a childhood-onset chronic condition implies that children do not only have to cope with their condition and its consequences for their daily life, but also need to reach various developmental milestones while passing through childhood, early adolescence, late adolescence and eventually attaining young adulthood. Young people are, for example, expected to leave their parents' or caregivers' homes eventually, pursue educational and vocational or professional careers, start their own families and thus, as autonomous adults, they are expected to participate and fulfill meaningful roles in society. This multifaceted life-stage transition to adulthood is already challenging but is extra demanding for those with (childhood-onset) chronic conditions [2]. These young people have to balance the usual developmental tasks of growing up with additional adaptive tasks related to their chronic condition. Fulfillment of these tasks is important for adjustment to adult life [3]. Moos and Holahan [4] described the following adaptive tasks for people with chronic conditions: managing symptoms, managing treatment, forming relationships with health care providers, managing emotions, maintaining a positive self-image, relating to family members and friends and preparing for an uncertain future

J. N. T. Sattoe (✉) · A. van Staa
Research Center Innovations in Care, Rotterdam University of Applied Sciences,
Rotterdam, The Netherlands
e-mail: j.n.t.sattoe@hr.nl

© Springer Nature Switzerland AG 2021   37
J. N. T. Sattoe et al. (eds.), *Self-Management of Young People with Chronic
Conditions*, https://doi.org/10.1007/978-3-030-64293-8_3

[4]. Note that these tasks relate to the medical, role and emotional domains of self-management [5], and require specific self-management skills (see also Table 3.1). Balancing and navigating between normal developmental and additional adaptive tasks related to the chronic condition is complex. A chronic condition and its treatment can have manifold effects on development and daily life, while at the same time developmental changes can affect both the condition and its treatment [7–9].

3.2   Growing Up with a Childhood-Onset Chronic Condition

Growth, physical appearance, relationships with relatives and peers, social participation and emotional wellbeing may all be influenced by a chronic condition [8–11]. Several studies showed that young people with chronic conditions reach developmental milestones later and are at risk for less favourable psychosocial development compared to their healthy peers [12, 13]. Adolescents confirm that having a chronic condition complicates school participation and the development of friendships through frequent hospitalizations and disclosure issues [14]. Mental health is often compromised as well. Young people with chronic conditions report elevated levels of anxiety and depressive symptoms and lower self-esteem compared to healthy peers [15–17]. On the other hand, usual developmental changes, like the onset of puberty, may negatively influence disease patterns and symptoms. Hormones may for example negatively impact disease parameters like growth hormone does for blood values in diabetes [8]. Young people are reported to have poorer disease control than other age groups, and to show problem behaviours or risk-taking behaviours [8, 18, 19], complicating management of the condition and its treatment. Another change young people have to deal with is the transfer from paediatric to adult care. Suboptimal transfer may result in no-show in adult care or poor treatment adherence, accompanied by a risk of complications and deterioration of health [20]. Self-management in young people with chronic conditions is thus complicated by the reciprocal impact of transitioning to adulthood and having a chronic condition.

Furthermore, the additional adaptive tasks for people with chronic conditions require specific self-management skills that young people have to acquire while becoming adults. While doing so, they ideally and gradually take over the responsibility of caring for their chronic condition from their parents or caregivers. This initial dependency followed by a gradual shift in responsibility is also part of their development and unique to the case of young people with chronic conditions [21]. They, for instance, have to build up a relation with new healthcare professionals in adult care and have to engage in shared decision-making. Gall et al. [22] introduced the Shared Management Model (also see Chap. 8) in which they outline that, ideally, young people gradually transform from *receivers of care* to their own *managers or supervisors of care*. In this last stage, parents take on the role of consultants and healthcare professionals become resources instead of having the major responsibility [22]. The role of parents in this process is further highlighted in Chap. 6.

Table 3.1 Self-management tasks along the adaptive tasks of living with a chronic condition and the domains of self-management[a]

Self-management domains	Medical management	Role management	Emotional management
Adaptive tasks of living with a chronic condition			
Managing symptoms and treatment	• Understanding: the disease; (the necessity of) medication and treatment regimen; and side effects • Use of specific treatment devices or techniques • Dealing with symptoms • Self-monitoring of clinical outcomes • Drafting an individualized care plan • Knowing where to find information about the disease • Knowing about the risks of risk behaviours (e.g. alcohol abuse).		
Forming relationships with healthcare professionals	• Accessing healthcare • Communication with healthcare professionals • Managing doctor visits • Coping with hospitalizations • Knowing when to ask for medical help • Having organizational skills		
Relating to family members and friends	• Child–parent sharing/ teamwork	• Social initiation and friendship making; having a social network; maintaining family and romantic relationships (sexuality)	
	• Knowing when to ask for (medical) help	• Participating in normal social activities; keeping up with peers (e.g. via internet or social media) • Disclosure (educating peers) • Communication and social problem-solving	

(continued)

Table 3.1 (continued)

Self-management domains	Medical management	Role management	Emotional management
Preparing for an uncertain future	• Setting goals for healthcare transition	• Setting goals and having dreams for the future related to school, work, community, living, housing, recreation and leisure	
		• Setting life goals	
		• Independent living	
		• Traveling/staying abroad	
		• Having organizational skills	
Managing emotions			• Dealing with fear-related thinking
			• Sharing feelings and experiences, also feelings related to the condition
			• Accepting the condition
			• Healthy expressions of anger and transforming or managing anger
			• Stress management; having helpful positive thoughts
			• Managing the impact of or decreasing negative thoughts
			• Spirituality
Maintaining a positive self-image			• Self-confidence/ self-esteem building
			• Developing a positive body image/body esteem
			• Building self-efficacy/ self-appreciation

[a]Adapted with permission from Sattoe et al. [6]

Taking up an active role in healthcare is not self-evident for young people. While adolescents want to be involved as equal partners in their care, this wish often remains unfulfilled in daily practice. During consultations, they mostly act like bystanders because their participation is not requested, nor encouraged [23, 24]. Also, preferences of young people often are not met by their actual experiences, which can have negative emotional consequences [25]. This difficulty in becoming independent and gaining autonomy is also present outside healthcare. A qualitative study comparing the views of adolescents and their parents, showed that life beliefs of young people and their parents can clash, leading to child–parent conflict [26] and resulting in negative outcomes regarding lived experiences, social participation, and the overall transition to adulthood [27, 28]. A recent review focusing on how children assume self-management responsibility from their parents showed that this includes a complex process that is influenced by multiple contextual factors [29]. Self-management in young people with chronic conditions is thus complicated by the shift from dependency to independency.

The developmental context of young people with chronic conditions hence impacts self-management and that is why self-management should be seen as transitional process [30] that is inevitably linked to their overall transition to adulthood [3]. Also, while the challenges are manifold, young people are generally motivated and confident about their ability to learn new skills. They often embrace the prospect of becoming autonomous adults, and many have an optimistic outlook on the future [2].

3.3   Frameworks for Self-Management and Self-Management Support of Young People

There are different frameworks that may be useful in addressing the challenges of self-management in young people with chronic conditions. A general framework that is often linked to self-management is the World Health Organization's International Classification of Functioning, Disability and Health (ICF; Fig. 3.1) [31]. While the ICF is not specifically designed for use in case of young people, it has been applied successfully to young people with chronic conditions in various

Fig. 3.1 International classification of functioning, disability and health

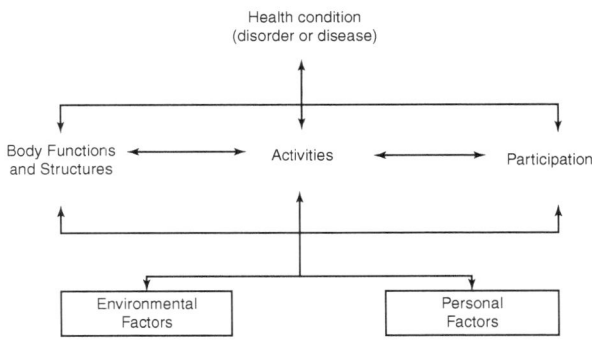

studies [21, 32–35]. The ICF is a biopsychosocial model that pretends to combine both the medical model of disease and the social model of disability. It considers three core components of functioning, i.e. body functions, activity and participation, within the sphere of an individual's health condition and contextual factors (environmental and personal factors). The ICF emphasizes the importance of *capacity* and *performance* in functioning. Capacity refers to the ability of a person to complete a task or action in a standard environment, while performance refers to performing this task or action in his or her own environment [31]. Regarding self-management of young people, the gaps between capacity and performance may help professionals (and others) to understand the support needs of these young people [21]. The ICF presumes that by addressing these barriers, functioning can be improved. Although the presence of mutual influences of an individual's health condition and context on daily functioning is described in the model, the ICF remains a general framework that does not specify self-management processes and tasks and the context in which self-management takes place. Also, the ICF has been criticized for being normative and not paying enough attention to people's lived experiences and the enhancement of their agency [36].

A more specific framework is the conceptual model of Modi et al. named the Paediatric Self-management Model (PSM) [37]. The PSM is a socio-ecological model that embeds self-management behaviours of young people with chronic conditions within four different domains: individual, family, community, and healthcare system. The underlying notion is that modifiable and non-modifiable factors in each domain determine self-management behaviours through cognitive, emotional and social processes. These self-management behaviours affect adherence and so influence outcomes (at both individual and system level) [37]. In this context, adherence is defined as "the extent to which a person's behaviour coincides with medical or health advice" [37]. The importance given to adherence as a mediating construct shows that the PSM focuses on medical treatment (outcomes). The developers mention that "self-management behaviours, which are conducted by a child or family member, are performed in the context of care for the chronic condition. This does not assume positive or negative impact, only that the behaviour was conducted for the purpose of treatment" [37]. The assumption that self-management behaviours are solely conducted for the purpose of treatment, however, does not concur with the holistic view on self-management.

The shifting importance of the medical, role and emotional domains is emphasized in the Self-management Support Model for Young People (SSMYP; Fig. 3.2) [3]. The SSMYP does not elaborate on specific self-management processes and outcomes, but tries to depict the unique context of young people growing up with chronic conditions and their specific self-management challenges. The SSMYP conceptualizes self-management as a dynamic process that requires flexibility in shifting between different *content* (the domains of self-management) and *roles* (of the people involved) [3]. The interaction between healthcare professionals and young people is shown as a continuum of directivity, acknowledging that sometimes professionals will take the lead and sometimes patients will—and that young people will have to learn forming partnerships with their healthcare professionals. The

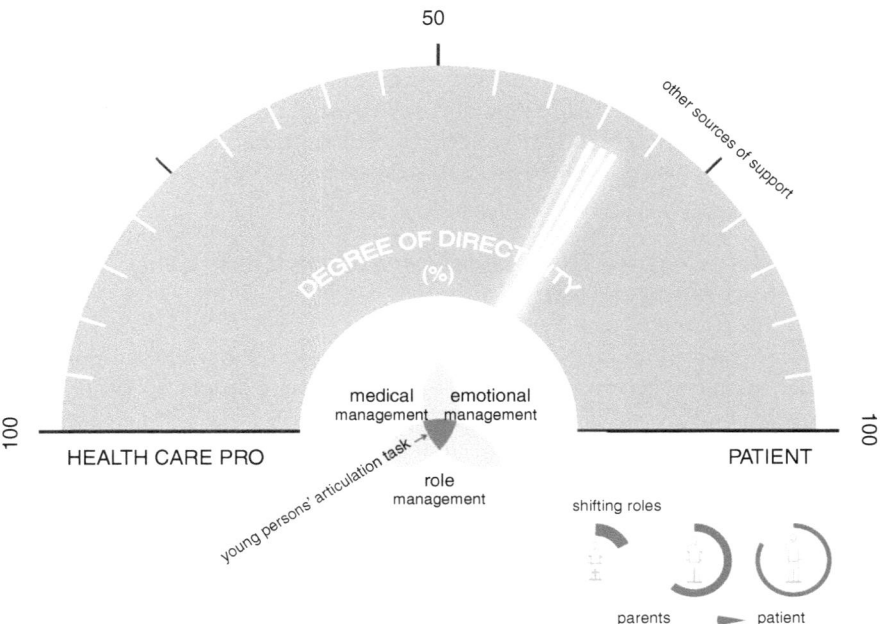

Fig. 3.2 Self-management support model for young people. (Sattoe, J.N.T. (2015). Growing up with a Chronic Condition: Challenges for Self-management and Self-management Support. Rotterdam: Erasmus University Rotterdam. ISBN: 978-94-6169-684-7)

(development of the) patient–provider relationship will be further explored in Chap. 5. The model also points towards shifting roles and autonomy of youth and their parents, which will be further explored in Chap. 6; and the fact that support may also come for others as is the case in peer support, as will be elaborated upon in Chap. 7. Finally, the SSMYP mentions an "articulating task" for young people when shifting between domains of self-management. This has to do with the inter-relatedness of the medical, role and emotional domains. Young people have to learn how to coordinate the tasks and priorities related to each domain within their capac-ities, this articulating task is the core of self-management [3].

The ICF, PSM and SSMYP are different models that may be seen as complemen-tary to each other. Still, there are some similarities between the models that may further enhance our understanding of self-management of young people with chronic conditions. First, all three conceptualize self-management as a dynamic process rather than a fixed ability. This is in line with seeing self-management of young people with chronic conditions as a "transitional process" [30]. Second, the ICF and the SSMYP both endorse a biopsychosocial view, underlining the impor-tant of all three domains of self-management. Finally, the ICF and the PSM both emphasize that self-management is influenced by contextual factors and all three models recognize the importance of others (e.g. parents, family, friends) in the pro-cess. There are also some points raised by the different models individually that deserve further exploration. First, the ICF distinguished the constructs of capacity and performance. Second, the PSM emphasizes that factors influencing self-management processes (and ultimately behaviour) can be either modifiable or unmodifiable. Third, the SSMYP points towards articulation work as the core self-management task. Before further exploration of these points, we review the theories and theoretical constructs underlying self-management.

3.4   Theories and Theoretical Constructs Underlying Self-Management

The theory that is most often linked to self-management is the social learning theory or social cognitive theory of Bandura [38], both in young people [6, 39, 40] and in adults with chronic conditions [41–44]. This theory implies that self-management is something that (young) people learn through information given by others (social persuasion by an authority), by observing others (social modelling) and by trial and error (mastery experiences). An important construct in the social cognitive theory of Bandura is self-efficacy. Self-efficacy refers to an individual's belief in his or her capacity to execute and control over certain tasks [45]. The idea is that higher self-efficacy will lead to "better" self-management, and that self-management interventions (SMI) should foster self-efficacy [44]. Often, instead of referring to the theory, studies use individual theoretical constructs to inform SMI [39, 41]. In this light, self-efficacy is often related to self-management [5, 46] and used as an outcome in the evaluation of SMI [6].

Another theory that is regularly linked to self-management is the theory of self-regulation. Again, this is both in young people [6, 39] and in adults with chronic conditions [42]. This theory is generally labelled as the self-regulation theory, but some more specifically refer to Bandura's social cognitive theory of self-regulation. The main idea is that people self-regulate to achieve previously set goals. Goals-setting is thus an important aspect of the theory, and Bandura [38] mentions three elements of self-regulation: (1) self-monitoring (of behaviour, its determinants and its outcomes), (2) judgement of the behaviour considering the context (e.g. is this behaviour in this context beneficial for me?), and (3) affective self-reaction (e.g. problem-solving) [38]. Barlow and colleagues (2002, p. 178) describe self-management as "… to monitor one's condition and to effect the cognitive, behavioural and emotional responses necessary to maintain a satisfactory quality of life" and define self-management as "a dynamic and continuous process of self-regulation…". The construct of self-efficacy is also seen as an important mechanism in the self-regulation theory [38]. Whereas self-regulation is more like the strategy to achieve pre-set goals, self-efficacy refers to the extent to which people think they will succeed in achieving these goals.

Another construct that is essential in the self-regulation theory is "self-determination", which is defined as "a combination of skills, knowledge, and beliefs that enable a person to engage in goal-directed, self-regulated, autonomous behaviour" [47]. The last part of this definition emphasizes that self-determination has to do with individual agency, e.g. having own priorities and making own decisions.

Apart from a construct, self-determination is also mentioned as a theory in itself. The self-determination theory emphasizes three basic needs: (1) having a sense of personal competence, (2) social relatedness (e.g. good relationships with others) and (3) autonomy [48, 49]. These are all line with self-management. Notable is that self-efficacy, again, seems to be an important construct (although not explicitly mentioned as such). Summarizing, all the mentioned theories show that self-efficacy, competency, social context and relatedness, and autonomy determine how young people perform self-management. We now explore the specific tasks and skills required for learning how to self-manage, the influencing factors, and self-management interventions.

3.5 Self-Management Tasks of Young People and Required Skills

Self-management of people with chronic conditions is about living with a chronic condition and thus is a lifetime task [50]. Each domain of self-management comes with its own adaptive tasks and required corresponding skills. For young people, the uptake of these tasks is extra challenging because they have to deal with additional developmental tasks that may interfere or even overlap with their self-management tasks [3]. Also, young people have less (life) experience than older adults which can make self-management more challenging. Therefore, they have a wider range of self-management tasks than adults [37]. Yet, literature on what these self-management tasks of young people entail is scarce.

In adults with chronic conditions, Schulman-Green et al. [51] specify processes, tasks and skills of self-management [51]. The list is long and self-management tasks evolve around the chronic condition and health needs, navigating healthcare, spirituality and social roles, and emotional adjustment. Corresponding skills vary from general life skills like "carrying out normal tasks and responsibilities" or "advocating for self" to specific skills like "monitoring and managing symptoms" and "coordinating services/appointments and insurance" [51].

In a systematic overview of SMI for young people with chronic conditions, the content of these interventions was reviewed [6]. This gives insight into what is seen as important for young people to learn to self-manage their chronic condition. In Table 3.1, we present it alongside the domains of self-management and the adaptive tasks of living with a chronic condition as described by Moos and Holahan [4]: managing symptoms, managing treatment, forming relationships with healthcare professionals, managing emotions, maintaining a positive self-image, relating to family members and friends and preparing for an uncertain future.

Another recent review of interventions for young people with chronic conditions has found similar content of interventions [52]. Corresponding self-management skills are problem-solving skills, decision-making skills, resource utilization skills, social and communication skills and goal setting skills [5, 52]. On top of these comes the articulation task, which Lorig and Holman [5] describe as the core self-management skill of "self-tailoring" [5], i.e. using one's skills to know and prioritize needs (and act accordingly). Required self-management skills are summarized in Table 3.2.

Table 3.2 Required self-management skills

Skills	In relation to self-management
Problem-solving	Solving problems by assessing situations and finding appropriate solutions
Decision-making	Being able to make the right decisions on the right time and in the right order
Resource utilization	Knowing when and how to utilize resources like finding and using the right information; and being able to involve others in time
Social relations and communication	Managing relationships with healthcare professionals: being an active partner in healthcare, reporting changes in health and discussing these with healthcare professionals, and being able to make argued decisions and share these with healthcare professionals
Goal setting	Being able to set goals and make a realistic planning to achieve these goals; also, being able to go from planning to practicing
Articulation or self-tailoring	Monitoring the course of disease, being able to prioritize accordingly, being flexible, and initiate timely adjustment when needed

3.6   Factors That Influence Self-Management of Young People

Different factors can influence self-management of young people with chronic conditions. Modi and colleagues [37] visualized that these can be both modifiable and non-modifiable and can operate at different levels: the individual level, the family level, the community level and the healthcare system level. In a review of barriers and facilitators of self-management among young people with chronic conditions different influencing factors were found [53], as well as in other studies [54–59]. These are summarized in Table 3.3 and placed alongside the categorisation and levels mentioned in the PSM. To complete the list the extra level "chronic condition" was added.

At the individual level, modifiable factors mostly cover the way young people see themselves and if they feel competent enough to manage their condition. Most factors can influence self-management both negatively and positively. Wanting to lead a "normal" life for instance, can be a motivation for some young people, while at the same time it can create pressure for others. Findings about the influence of non-modifiable personal factors are mostly mixed and thus unclear [53]. Parental involvement in self-management can as well be both positive and negative for young people. If parents leave room for young people to develop autonomy and eventually grow independent, this is beneficial. On the other hand, if they worry about letting go and want to force their own involvement upon their child's life, it often creates child–parent conflicts, complicating self-management. Similarly, relationships with peers and teachers can be supportive or not. This is likely also true for relationships with colleagues and supervisors in the work environment. Finally, on the healthcare system level, relationships with providers, perception of ownership of care and shared management can be important. Financial costs and difficult treatment regimens can complicate self-management. The list of influencing factors in Table 3.3 is not exhaustive and it is noteworthy

Table 3.3 Factors that influence self-management of young people

	Modifiable	Non-modifiable
Individual	Self-concept (normalization)	Age
	Health beliefs	Gender
	Self-efficacy	Intrapersonal characteristics, e.g. intellectual/cognitive capacity
	Knowledge (about the chronic condition)	
	Feeling of autonomy	
	Problem-solving skills	
	Psychosocial functioning	
Family	Parental involvement and support in self-management	Socioeconomic status
	Parental attitudes towards chronic condition	Ethnicity/culture
		Marital status of parents
Community	Peer relationships/support	Social stigma
	Interactions with teachers (e.g. understanding of teachers)	
Healthcare system	Support by healthcare providers	Financial costs
	Patient–provider relationship	Access to healthcare
	Shared management with providers and parents	
	Ownership of care	
Chronic condition	Attitude towards condition	Visibility
	(Complicated) regimen/treatment	Age at onset of condition
		Predictability
		Complicated regimen/treatment

that most studies into influencing factors and experiences of young people only included adolescents. Studies about young adults are scarce. Also, little is known about the interaction between different factors.

3.7   Self-Management Interventions

A wide variety of SMI exist for young people with different chronic conditions [6], although the self-management challenges are similar across conditions [40]. Most individual intervention studies are conducted in the United States [6, 52], focus on a particular diagnosis with asthma and diabetes on top of the list [6, 39, 40, 52], and are conducted in young people in the age from 12 to 18 year old [6]. Interventions aim at different areas of self-management. Eighty-one SMI for young people (7–25 years) were reviewed, and most SMI solely aimed at medical management, while very few consider emotional management [6, 60]. This finding is in contrast with the notion that self-management is a broad concept and encompasses more than medical management and indicates that the translation from theory to practice is slow. Yet, a shift seems to be noticeable. In an update of the review (see Chap. 4), we found new interventions aiming at emotional management, while no new interventions were included that were solely targeted at medical management.

Regarding the format, SMI can be applied at individual level or group level and sometimes parents of young people with chronic conditions also participate in interventions. Formats include among others educational sessions, skills training sessions, motivational interviewing sessions, cognitive behavioural therapy sessions, family sessions, telemedicine systems, peer support activities and art therapy sessions [6, 52]. Saxby et al. [40] recommended eight key educational components for SMI (regardless of the format): structured and sequenced curricula, reinforcement, active participation, collaboration, autonomy, feedback, multiple exposures and problem-solving [40]. These seem appropriate as they link to the theoretical assumptions underlying self-management. Professionals that facilitate self-management support are, among others, trained interventionists, nurses, clinicians, psychologists and therapists, and can also include whole healthcare teams [6, 52]. The setting of interventions also varies. While they are mostly conducted in outpatient clinics of hospitals, they can also take place at home, schools, public environments, and online [6, 52].

3.8   Evaluation and Outcomes of Self-Management Interventions

As the types and content of SMI vary, so do the outcome measures used in evaluation studies [6, 39, 52, 61]. Studies for instance measure adherence, disease knowledge, clinical outcomes, self-efficacy, quality of life, self-management skills and behaviours. Although this could logically be attributed to the different areas interventions focus on, mismatches between content of interventions and outcome measures used in evaluation studies are not uncommon [6]. This hampers conclusions about the effectiveness of SMI for young people with chronic conditions in meta-analyses [3].

The uncritical use of outcome measures was also mentioned by others, and the establishment of a core set of measurement instruments for SMI is recommended [61–63]. So far, we only found one study that identified a core outcome set for clinical trials of interventions for young adults with type 1 diabetes. Eight outcomes were recommended: (1) measures of diabetes-related stress, (2) diabetes-related quality of life, (3) number of severe hypoglycaemic events, (4) self-management behaviour, (5) number of instances of diabetic ketoacidosis (DKA), (6) objectively measured glycated haemoglobin (HbA1C), (7) level of clinic engagement, and (8) perceived level of control over diabetes [64]. Both medical and emotional management seem to be covered in these, but role management is not. An outcome measure related to role management could be the Rotterdam Transition Profile, that measures the attainment of independence in areas such as education, work, independent living, sexuality and intimate relations, etc. [65, 66].

Predefined outcome sets do not exist. One could also wonder whether it would be feasible and helpful to define core outcomes for every diagnosis separately.

Therefore, current studies would benefit from a more systematic approach to the evaluation of SMI. Steps in such an approach could be [3]:

1. Review the content of interventions: Which domains of self-management are targeted?
2. Establish content-related criteria for the selection of participants: Who needs the intervention?
3. Select theory- and content-related outcome measures: What is expected to change?
4. Decide on measurement instruments: Disease-specific or generic?

Despite the heterogeneity in interventions and outcome measures used and the methodological limitations of evaluation studies, some evidence on the effectiveness of SMI for young people with chronic conditions has been extracted in recent reviews. This will be reviewed in the next chapter.

3.9 Key Recommendations

• Acknowledge that balancing and navigating between normal developmental and additional adaptive tasks related to the chronic condition, is complex for young people and parents alike.
• Be aware that growth, physical appearance, relationships with relatives and peers, social participation, and emotional wellbeing may all be influenced by the chronic condition and that being "different" may cause additional emotional strain on young people.
• View the development of self-management skills as a necessary prerequisite for an optimal transfer from paediatric to adult care. It is an intrinsic part of transitioning to adulthood and to adult care.
• Include parents or caregivers in the process of building self-management skills, as young people gradually need to take over the responsibility of caring for their chronic condition from them.
• Involve children and adolescents in all healthcare-related decisions and encourage that they participate in their healthcare as much as possible.
• Use holistic, biopsychosocial models to describe self-management tasks and do not only focus on the medical domain and tasks.
• Self-efficacy is an important determinant of self-management. Therefore, facilitate environments that allow young people to learn from others and to gain mastery experiences.
• In developing self-management interventions for young people with chronic conditions, both disease-specific and generic self-management tasks should be addressed.
• Use theory to build self-management interventions and use a systematic approach for the evaluation.

- Make sure that the selected outcomes in the evaluation of self-management interventions match both the goal and the content of the intervention.
- Be aware that there is no "one size fits all" approach, as the development of self-management is a dynamic and individualized process.

3.10   Conclusion

Growing up with a childhood-onset chronic condition implies that young people do not only have to cope with their condition and its consequences in daily life, but also need to reach various developmental milestones in order to achieve autonomy in adulthood. Learning to perform self-management tasks is a challenge for young people, their families, and healthcare professionals alike. This is a complex process that requires flexibility, trust, and support on the part of parents and professionals so that adolescents can build self-confidence and enhance their self-efficacy. The development of self-management is influenced by many factors, both on the level of the individual, the family, the community and the healthcare system. Self-management does not only involve medical tasks, but also involves managing the psychological and social consequences of living with a chronic condition. Self-management skills are often complex and include problem-solving, decision-making, resource utilization, building social relations, goal setting and self-tailoring. Many of such adaptive tasks are not disease-specific but represent generic challenges. Still, at present, most interventions aiming at enhancing self-management skills in young people only target medical management skills. Very few focus on the emotional trials that are inherent to living with chronic conditions. Furthermore, the evaluation of self-management interventions is often comprised by the fact that there seems to be little consensus on suitable outcomes.

Adolescence is often described as a stormy period with multiple transitions in various life domains. Still, young people themselves generally have an optimistic view of the future and embrace the possibilities of adulthood. This offers healthcare professionals and parents the opportunity to empower young people in their journey towards adulthood. Self-management does not imply doing it all by yourself; but it starts with the acknowledgement of the right and the need to include young people in (decisions about) their own care and life.

References

1. Barlow J, Wright C, Sheasby J, Turner A, Hainsworth J. Self-management approaches for people with chronic conditions: a review. Patient Educ Couns. 2002;48(2):177–87. https://doi.org/10.1016/s0738-3991(02)00032-0.
2. van Staa A. On your own feet: adolescents with chronic conditions and their preferences and competencies for care (Dissertation). Rotterdam: Erasmus University Rotterdam; 2012. (ISBN 978-90-79059-03-4).
3. Sattoe JNT. Growing up with a chronic condition: challenges for self-management and self-management support (Dissertation). Rotterdam: Erasmus University Rotterdam; 2015. (ISBN 978-94-6169-684-7).

4. Moos RH, Holahan CJ. Adaptive tasks and methods of coping with illness and disability. In: Coping with chronic illness and disability. New York, NY: Springer; 2007. p. 107–26. https://doi.org/10.1007/978-0-387-48670-3_6.
5. Lorig KR, Holman HR. Self-management education: history, definition, outcomes, and mechanisms. Ann Behav Med. 2003;26(1):1–7. https://doi.org/10.1207/S15324796ABM2601_01.
6. Sattoe JNT, Bal MI, Roelofs PD, Bal R, Miedema HS, van Staa A. Self-management interventions for young people with chronic conditions: a systematic overview. Patient Educ Couns. 2015;98(6):704–15. https://doi.org/10.1016/j.pec.2015.03.004.
7. Sawyer SM, Drew S, Yeo MS, Britto MT. Adolescents with a chronic condition: challenges living, challenges treating. Lancet. 2007;369(9571):1481–9. https://doi.org/10.1016/S0140-6736(07)60370-5.
8. Suris J-C, Michaud P-A, Viner R. The adolescent with a chronic condition. Part I: developmental issues. Arch Dis Child. 2004;89(10):938–42. https://doi.org/10.1136/adc.2003.045369.
9. Yeo M, Sawyer S. Chronic illness and disability. BMJ. 2005;330(7493):721–3. https://doi.org/10.1136/bmj.330.7493.721.
10. Ferro MA. Adolescents and young adults with physical illness: a comparative study of psychological distress. Acta Paediatr. 2014;103(1):e32–7. https://doi.org/10.1111/apa.12429.
11. Gorter JW, Stewart D, Smith MW, King G, Wright M, Nguyen T, et al. Pathways toward positive psychosocial outcomes and mental health for youth with disabilities: a knowledge synthesis of developmental trajectories. Can J Commun Ment Health. 2014;33(1):45–61. https://doi.org/10.7870/cjcmh-2014-005.
12. Maurice-Stam H, Nijhof SL, Monninkhof AS, Heymans HS, Grootenhuis MA. Review about the impact of growing up with a chronic disease showed delays achieving psychosocial milestones. Acta Paediatr. 2019;108:2157. https://doi.org/10.1111/apa.14918.
13. Pinquart M, Teubert D. Academic, physical, and social functioning of children and adolescents with chronic physical illness: a meta-analysis. J Pediatr Psychol. 2011;37(4):376–89. https://doi.org/10.1093/jpepsy/jsr106.
14. Taylor RM, Gibson F, Franck LS. The experience of living with a chronic illness during adolescence: a critical review of the literature. J Clin Nurs. 2008;17(23):3083–91. https://doi.org/10.1111/j.1365-2702.2008.02629.x.
15. Pinquart M, Shen Y. Depressive symptoms in children and adolescents with chronic physical illness: an updated meta-analysis. J Pediatr Psychol. 2010;36(4):375–84. https://doi.org/10.1093/jpepsy/jsq104.
16. Pinquart M, Shen Y. Anxiety in children and adolescents with chronic physical illnesses: a meta-analysis. Acta Paediatr. 2011a;100(8):1069–76. https://doi.org/10.1111/j.1651-2227.2011.02223.x.
17. Pinquart M. Self-esteem of children and adolescents with chronic illness: a meta-analysis. Child Care Health Dev. 2013;39(2):153–61. https://doi.org/10.1111/j.1365-2214.2012.01397.x.
18. Michaud P, Suris J, Viner R. The adolescent with a chronic condition. Part II: healthcare provision. Arch Dis Child. 2004;89(10):943–9. https://doi.org/10.1136/adc.2003.045377.
19. Pinquart M, Shen Y. Behavior problems in children and adolescents with chronic physical illness: a meta-analysis. J Pediatr Psychol. 2011b;36(9):1003–16. https://doi.org/10.1093/jpepsy/jsr042.
20. Lugasi T, Achille M, Stevenson M. Patients' perspective on factors that facilitate transition from child-centered to adult-centered health care: a theory integrated metasummary of quantitative and qualitative studies. J Adolesc Health. 2011;48(5):429–40. https://doi.org/10.1016/j.jadohealth.2010.10.016.
21. Lozano P, Houtrow A. Supporting self-management in children and adolescents with complex chronic conditions. Pediatrics. 2018;141(Suppl 3):S233–41. https://doi.org/10.1542/peds.2017-1284H.
22. Gall C, Kingsnorth S, Healy H. Growing up ready: a shared management approach. Phys Occup Ther Pediatr. 2006;26(4):47–62. https://doi.org/10.1080/J006v26n04_04.
23. Coyne I. Children's participation in consultations and decision-making at health service level: a review of the literature. Int J Nurs Stud. 2008;45(11):1682–9. https://doi.org/10.1016/j.ijnurstu.2008.05.002.

24. van Staa A, On Your Own Feet Research Group. Unraveling triadic communication in hospital consultations with adolescents with chronic conditions: the added value of mixed methods research. Patient Educ Couns. 2011;82(3):455–64. https://doi.org/10.1016/j.pec.2010.12.001.
25. Jordan A, Wood F, Edwards A, Shepherd V, Joseph-Williams N. What adolescents living with long-term conditions say about being involved in decision-making about their healthcare: a systematic review and narrative synthesis of preferences and experiences. Patient Educ Couns. 2018;101(10):1725–35. https://doi.org/10.1016/j.pec.2018.06.006.
26. Peeters MA, Hilberink SR, van Staa A. The road to independence: lived experiences of youth with chronic conditions and their parents compared. J Pediatr Rehabil Med. 2014;7(1):33–42. https://doi.org/10.3233/PRM-140272.
27. Beresford B. On the road to nowhere? Young disabled people and transition. Child Care Health Dev. 2004;30(6):581–7. https://doi.org/10.1111/j.1365-2214.2004.00469.x.
28. Holmbeck GN, Johnson SZ, Wills KE, McKernon W, Rose B, Erklin S, Kemper T. Observed and perceived parental overprotection in relation to psychosocial adjustment in preadolescents with a physical disability: the mediational role of behavioral autonomy. J Consult Clin Psychol. 2002;70(1):96. https://doi.org/10.1037/0022-006X.70.1.96.
29. Nightingale R, McHugh G, Kirk S, Swallow V. Supporting children and young people to assume responsibility from their parents for the self-management of their long-term condition: an integrative review. Child Care Health Dev. 2019;45(2):175–88. https://doi.org/10.1111/cch.12645.
30. Ryan P, Sawin KJ. The individual and family self-management theory: background and perspectives on context, process, and outcomes. Nurs Outlook. 2009;57(4):217–225.e216. https://doi.org/10.1016/j.outlook.2008.10.004.
31. World Health Organization. International classification of functioning, disability and health: ICF. Geneva: World Health Organization; 2001.
32. Glader L, Plews-Ogan J, Agrawal R. Children with medical complexity: creating a framework for care based on the international classification of functioning, disability and health. Dev Med Child Neurol. 2016;58(11):1116–23. https://doi.org/10.1111/dmcn.13201.
33. Kraus de Camargo O. Systems of care: transition from the bio-psycho-social perspective of the international classification of functioning, disability and health. Child Care Health Dev. 2011;37(6):792–9. https://doi.org/10.1111/j.1365-2214.2011.01323.x.
34. McDougall J, Horgan K, Baldwin P, Tucker MA, Frid P. Employing the international classification of functioning, disability and health to enhance services for children and youth with chronic physical health conditions and disabilities. Paediatr Child Health. 2008;13(3):173–8. https://doi.org/10.1093/pch/13.3.173.
35. Nguyen T, Gorter J. Use of the international classification of functioning, disability and health as a framework for transition from paediatric to adult healthcare. Child Care Health Dev. 2014;40(6):759–61. https://doi.org/10.1111/cch.12125.
36. Mitra S, Shakespeare T. Remodeling the ICF. Remodeling the ICF. Disabil Health J. 2019;12:337–9. https://doi.org/10.1016/j.dhjo.2019.01.008.
37. Modi AC, Pai AL, Hommel KA, Hood KK, Cortina S, Hilliard ME, et al. Pediatric self-management: a framework for research, practice, and policy. Pediatrics. 2012;129(2):e473–85. https://doi.org/10.1542/peds.2011-1635.
38. Bandura A. Social cognitive theory of self-regulation. Organ Behav Hum Decis Process. 1991;50(2):248–87.
39. Ng CY, Thomas-Uribe M, Yang YA, Chu MC, Liu S-D, Pulendran UP, et al. Theory-based health behavior interventions for pediatric chronic disease management: a systematic review. JAMA Pediatr. 2018;172(12):1177–86. https://doi.org/10.1001/jamapediatrics.2018.3039.
40. Saxby N, Beggs S, Battersby M, Lawn S. What are the components of effective chronic condition self-management education interventions for children with asthma, cystic fibrosis, and diabetes? A systematic review. Patient Educ Couns. 2019;102:607–22. https://doi.org/10.1016/j.pec.2018.11.001.
41. Miller WR, Lasiter S, Ellis RB, Buelow JM. Chronic disease self-management: a hybrid concept analysis. Nurs Outlook. 2015;63(2):154–61. https://doi.org/10.1016/j.outlook.2014.07.005.

42. Moore SM, Schiffman R, Waldrop-Valverde D, Redeker NS, McCloskey DJ, Kim MT, et al. Recommendations of common data elements to advance the science of self-management of chronic conditions. J Nurs Scholarsh. 2016;48(5):437–47. https://doi.org/10.1111/jnu.12233.

43. Packer TL, Fracini A, Audulv Å, Alizadeh N, van Gaal BG, Warner G, Kephart G. What we know about the purpose, theoretical foundation, scope and dimensionality of existing self-management measurement tools: a scoping review. Patient Educ Couns. 2018;101(4):579–95. https://doi.org/10.1016/j.pec.2017.10.014.

44. Richardson J, Loyola-Sanchez A, Sinclair S, Harris J, Letts L, MacIntyre NJ, et al. Self-management interventions for chronic disease: a systematic scoping review. Clin Rehabil. 2014;28(11):1067–77. https://doi.org/10.1177/0269215514532478.

45. Bandura A. Self-efficacy: the exercise of control. New York, NY: W.H. Freeman and Company; 1997.

46. Ong BN, Rogers A, Kennedy A, Bower P, Sanders T, Morden A, et al. Behaviour change and social blinkers? The role of sociology in trials of self-management behaviour in chronic conditions. Sociol Health Illn. 2014;36(2):226–38. https://doi.org/10.1111/1467-9566.12113.

47. Field S, Martin J, Miller R, Ward M, Wehmeyer M. A practical guide for teaching self-determination: ERIC; 1998.

48. Deci EL, Ryan RM. The "what" and "why" of goal pursuits: human needs and the self-determination of behavior. Psychol Inq. 2000;11(4):227–68. https://doi.org/10.1207/S15327965PLI1104_01.

49. Ryan RM, Deci EL. Self-determination theory and the facilitation of intrinsic motivation, social development, and well-being. Am Psychol. 2000;55(1):68. https://doi.org/10.1037/0003-066X.55.1.68.

50. Van de Velde D, De Zutter F, Satink T, Costa U, Janquart S, Senn D, De Vriendt P. Delineating the concept of self-management in chronic conditions: a concept analysis. BMJ Open. 2019;9(7):e027775. https://doi.org/10.1136/bmjopen-2018-027775.

51. Schulman-Green D, Jaser S, Martin F, Alonzo A, Grey M, McCorkle R, et al. Processes of self-management in chronic illness. J Nurs Scholarsh. 2012;44(2):136–44. https://doi.org/10.1111/j.1547-5069.2012.01444.x.

52. Stenberg U, Haaland-Øverby M, Koricho AT, Trollvik A, Kristoffersen LGR, Dybvig S, Vågan A. How can we support children, adolescents and young adults in managing chronic health challenges? A scoping review on the effects of patient education interventions. Health Expect. 2019;22(5):849–62. https://doi.org/10.1111/hex.12906.

53. Lindsay S, Kingsnorth S, Hamdani Y. Barriers and facilitators of chronic illness self-management among adolescents: a review and future directions. J Nurs Healthc Chronic Illn. 2011;3(3):186–208. https://doi.org/10.1111/j.1752-9824.2011.01090.x.

54. Holley S, Morris R, Knibb R, Latter S, Liossi C, Mitchell F, Roberts G. Barriers and facilitators to asthma self-management in adolescents: a systematic review of qualitative and quantitative studies. Pediatr Pulmonol. 2017;52(4):430–42. https://doi.org/10.1002/ppul.23556.

55. Lindsay S. A qualitative synthesis of adolescents' experiences of living with spina bifida. Qual Health Res. 2014;24(9):1298–309. https://doi.org/10.1177/1049732314546558.

56. Paine CW, Stollon NB, Lucas MS, Brumley LD, Poole ES, Peyton T, et al. Barriers and facilitators to successful transition from pediatric to adult inflammatory bowel disease care from the perspectives of providers. Inflamm Bowel Dis. 2014;20(11):2083–91. https://doi.org/10.1097/MIB.0000000000000136.

57. Schwartz L, Tuchman L, Hobbie W, Ginsberg J. A social-ecological model of readiness for transition to adult-oriented care for adolescents and young adults with chronic health conditions. Child Care Health Dev. 2011;37(6):883–95. https://doi.org/10.1111/j.1365-2214.2011.01282.x.

58. Stern A, Winning A, Ohanian D, Driscoll CFB, Starnes M, Glownia K, Holmbeck GN. Longitudinal associations between neuropsychological functioning and medical responsibility in youth with spina bifida: the moderational role of parenting behaviors. Child Neuropsychol. 2020;26:1026–46. https://doi.org/10.1080/09297049.2020.1751098.

59. Syed IA, Nathan PC, Barr R, Rosenberg-Yunger ZR, D'Agostino NM, Klassen AF. Examining factors associated with self-management skills in teenage survivors of cancer. J Cancer Surviv. 2016;10(4):686–91. https://doi.org/10.1007/s11764-016-0514-y.
60. Bal MI, Sattoe JNT, Roelofs PD, Bal R, van Staa A, Miedema HS. Exploring effectiveness and effective components of self-management interventions for young people with chronic physical conditions: a systematic review. Patient Educ Couns. 2016;99(8):1293–309. https://doi.org/10.1016/j.pec.2016.02.012.
61. Lindsay S, Kingsnorth S, Mcdougall C, Keating H. A systematic review of self-management interventions for children and youth with physical disabilities. Disabil Rehabil. 2014;36(4):276–88. https://doi.org/10.3109/09638288.2013.785605.
62. Nolte S, Elsworth GR, Newman S, Osborne RH. Measurement issues in the evaluation of chronic disease self-management programs. Qual Life Res. 2013;22(7):1655–64. https://doi.org/10.1007/s11136-012-0317-1.
63. Nolte S, Osborne RH. A systematic review of outcomes of chronic disease self-management interventions. Qual Life Res. 2013;22(7):1805–16. https://doi.org/10.1007/s11136-012-0302-8.
64. Byrne M, O'Connell A, Egan AM, Dinneen SF, Hynes L, O'Hara MC, et al. A core outcomes set for clinical trials of interventions for young adults with type 1 diabetes: an international, multi-perspective Delphi consensus study. Trials. 2017;18(1):602. https://doi.org/10.1186/s13063-017-2364-y.
65. Donkervoort M, Wiegerink DJ, Van Meeteren J, Stam HJ, Roebroeck ME, Netherlands, T. R. G. S. W. Transition to adulthood: validation of the Rotterdam Transition Profile for young adults with cerebral palsy and normal intelligence. Dev Med Child Neurol. 2009;51(1):53–62. https://doi.org/10.1111/j.1469-8749.2008.03115.x.
66. Zhang-Jiang S, Gorter JW. The use of the Rotterdam Transition Profile: 10 years in review. J Transit Med. 2018;1(1):20180002. https://doi.org/10.1515/jtm-2018-0002.

Exploring Components and Effects of Self-Management Interventions for Young People with Chronic Conditions

4

Marjolijn I. Bal, Jane N. T. Sattoe, Pepijn D. D. M. Roelofs, and AnneLoes van Staa

4.1   Introduction

It is important to help young people with chronic conditions to gradually develop self-management skills in all life areas, e.g., in work (intimate) relationships, sport activities, healthcare [1–3]. That is why self-management support is considered an integral part of healthcare [1–3]. It is often delivered using specific self-management interventions (SMI), and aims to help young people to (learn to) deal with the physical, emotional, and social consequences of their chronic condition in daily life.

Various studies evaluated SMI for young people with chronic conditions [1–8]. However, most of these studies are focused on specific diagnoses [4, 5, 8] while a non-categorical (i.e., generic) approach can be more helpful for practice [9, 10]. There are many similarities between young people with various chronic conditions, as they all face comparable challenges and adaptive tasks while growing up [11]. Also, components or elements of SMI are often similar across chronic conditions. A non-categorical approach to self-management could allow different healthcare teams to learn from each other, for instance by using similar intervention formats. Examples of such SMI are the Ready Steady Go and the Skills for Growing Up tools (see Chap. 8). Also, a non-categorical approach could stimulate the use of similar outcomes measures in evaluation studies, which would benefit research into effectiveness of SMI [11].

M. I. Bal (✉)
Research Center Innovations in Care, Rotterdam University of Applied Sciences, Rotterdam, The Netherlands

Department of Rehabilitation Medicine, Erasmus University Medical Center Rotterdam, Rotterdam, The Netherlands
e-mail: m.i.bal@hr.nl

J. N. T. Sattoe · P. D. D. M. Roelofs · A. van Staa
Research Center Innovations in Care, Rotterdam University of Applied Sciences, Rotterdam, The Netherlands

© Springer Nature Switzerland AG 2021   55
J. N. T. Sattoe et al. (eds.), *Self-Management of Young People with Chronic Conditions*, https://doi.org/10.1007/978-3-030-64293-8_4

This chapter presents an update of a systematic review of SMI for young persons with chronic conditions, employing a generic approach [12]. It elaborates on evidence of effectiveness of different outcome measures and provides insights into promising intervention components.

4.2 Systematic Literature Review

4.2.1 Searching for SMI

The search strategy consisted of variations and Boolean connections (AND, OR) of subject headings and keywords relating to self-management; children, adolescents, and young people; chronic illness/condition and physical disabilities and intervention [12]. Relevant variations of search terms were derived from database thesauruses and similar review articles. An information specialist helped define the final search strategy. Six databases were searched: Embase, Medline, PsycINFO, Web-of-Science, CINAHL, and Cochrane. Two researchers (MB, JS) independently completed the database searches by scrutinizing relevant reviews' references for additional relevant publications. Inclusion criteria for the studies found are presented in Table 4.1. In total, 10,939 studies were identified. Full texts of all agreed-upon articles ($n = 637$) were obtained. Then, two reviewers (MB, JS) independently decided on the inclusion of articles based on the full text, resulting in 69 publications (Fig. 4.1). The methodology checklists of the Scottish Intercollegiate Guidelines Network (SIGN) for randomized controlled trials [13] were used to assess their methodological quality.

4.2.2 Exploring Content and Components of SMI

Self-management support includes three domains: medical management (considering the treatment, symptoms, lifestyle, etc.), role management (considering social roles and participation), and emotional management (considering emotional consequences of having a chronic condition and emotional well-being) [14]. Next to the focus of SMI (i.e., which domain(s) of self-management do they address), data on several components of SMI were extracted: interventions' theoretical base; format

Table 4.1 Inclusion criteria

A	Study design: studies using a randomized controlled study design.
B	Study types: original research articles in English language published from January 2003–February 2019.
C	Interventions: studies focusing on the evaluation of SMI and describing the SMI or referring to previous description(s) of the intervention.
D	Outcome measures: studies considering clearly defined outcome measures.
E	Participants: studies focusing on young people aged 7–25 years with somatic chronic conditions or physical disabilities.

Fig. 4.1 Selection process

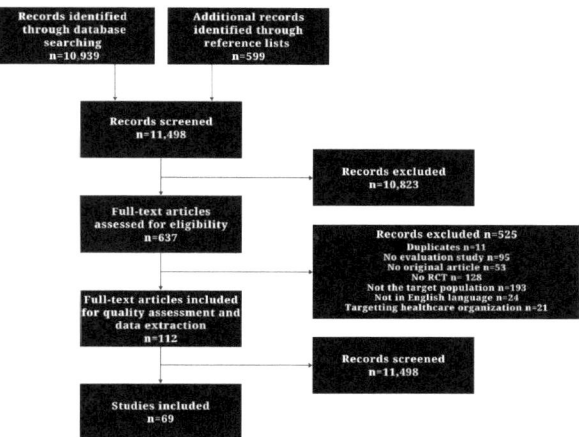

(group or individual or a combination of these); discipline (monodisciplinary or multidisciplinary); interventionists (e.g., psychologist or nurse); elements (e.g., education, peer-support, telemedicine); and setting (e.g., home, clinic, school).

4.2.3 Exploring Effectiveness and Effective Components

Two reviewers (MB, JS) independently clustered the specific study outcome measures into categories. GRADE was used to independently rate the overall quality of evidence for each category (see Appendix) [15].

Analyses to explore the effectiveness and the effective SMI components were performed for each outcome measure category separately. Random effects analysis was applied in which standardized mean differences between intervention and control group were calculated for each study [16]. In this way, effect sizes of statistically heterogeneous studies could be compared and an overview of effects on an outcome measured with different measurement instruments could be provided. Pooled estimates were not calculated, because interventions were clinically diverse (i.e., consisted of different intervention elements) and studies were methodologically diverse (i.e., different measurement instruments were used for evaluation).

In addition, to evaluate the effective intervention components, effect sizes of included studies that differed on particular intervention components were compared (regardless of the overall effects). A pattern of effects was only described when *at least* three studies were included and we used the cutoff point of two out of three studies (67%) as a minimum number of studies indicating effects in the same direction. If this last requirement could not be met, the pattern was described as showing no clear effects. Individual studies that showed a significant effect were weighted twice and individual studies that showed a trend (but not a significant effect) were weighted once.

4.3   Findings

In this chapter we included a total of 69 studies (27 additional studies compared to the original review) [17–85]. A description of study characteristics and intervention components per study is presented in Table 4.2.

4.3.1   SMI Components

4.3.1.1 Domains and Theories of Self-Management

More than half of the SMI solely targeted medical management (51%). Medical management was either disease-specific (e.g., self-monitoring of blood glucose values in diabetes) or consisted of more generic elements (e.g., making appointments in healthcare). One intervention only considered role management (2%) [67], referring to topics related to social participation, such as communication, assertiveness and keeping up with peers, while one intervention only considered emotional management (2%) [53], referring to young person's emotions and cognitions. Stress-management and relaxation techniques were discussed during this intervention program. Other SMI addressed multiple self-management domains: medical and emotion management (18%); medical and role management (12%); and medical, emotion, and role management (15%).

Most studies did not mention a theoretical base for the SMI (70%). When studies referred to a theory-driven framework, these included cognitive behavioral theory (14%), Bandura's (cognitive) social learning theory (6%), both cognitive behavioral theory and Bandura's (cognitive) social learning theory (3%), or other (7%).

4.3.1.2 Other Components

Interventions were applied at the individual level (61%), at group level (31%), or both (8%). The professional backgrounds of the interventionists were often not mentioned (45%). However, in the cases these were mentioned, SMI were mostly provided by one type of professional (monodisciplinary) (77%). Often a psychologist (27%) or a nurse (12%) was involved. Regarding intervention elements, SMI included: education (86%), cognitive restructuring (e.g., cognitive behavioral therapy) (24%), relaxation training (24%), peer-support (18%), discussion sessions (15%), telemedicine/e-health (using password protected websites with eLearning modules, written assignments, and/or games), phone calls by healthcare professionals or peers (15%), and training in problem-solving (14%), goal-setting (14%) or self-monitoring (e.g., keeping a diary with blood glucose values) (14%).

4.3.2   Outcomes of Self-Management Interventions

In general, results on effectiveness should be interpreted with some caution, because the quality of evidence for most outcome measures was low or very low (Appendix). This is mainly caused by the variability and heterogeneity of SMI. Also,

Table 4.2 Study characteristics and intervention components

Background		Participants		Study characteristics			Components of self-management interventions					
Studies	Country	Chronic condition	N	Methodological Quality[a]	Control	Outcome measure	Theoretical base (Yes)[b]	Domain of self-management[c]	Formats	Elements	Interventionists	Setting
Al-Sheyab et al. [85]	Jordan	Asthma	N = 261	Moderate	Usual care	Coping with the chronic condition in daily life	NA	MM	Group	Discussion	Peers	School
	Australia		I = 132			Disease knowledge				Education		
			C = 129			Quality of life				Problem-solving skills		
Ammerlaan et al. [17]	The Netherlands	Juvenile idiopathic arthritis	N = 67	Moderate	Usual care	Adherence	NA	MM + EM + RM	Group + individual	Communication skills	NA	Online
			I = 35			Coping with the chronic condition in daily life				Discussion		
						Quality of life				Education		
			C = 32			School attendance				Goal-setting skills		
										Peer-support		
Barakat et al. [44]	USA	Sickle cell disease	N = 37	Low	Another specific intervention	Coping with the chronic condition in daily life	NA	MM	Individual	Cognitive restructuring	Psychologist	Home
			I = 17			Disease knowledge				Education		
			C = 20			School attendance				Relaxation training		
						Symptoms				Self-monitoring		
Beebe et al. [45]	USA	Asthma	N = 22	Low	Waitlist	Psychological outcomes	NA	MM + EM	Group	Art-therapy	NA	School
						Quality of life				Discussion		
										Education		
										Problem-solving skills		

(continued)

Table 4.2 (continued)

	Background		Participants			Study characteristics				Components of self-management interventions					
Studies	Country		Chronic condition	N		Methodological Quality[a]	Control	Outcome measure	Theoretical base (Yes)[b]	Domain of self-management[c]	Formats	Elements	Interventionists	Setting
Behestipoor et al. [18]	Iran		Hemophilia	N = 40 / I = 20 / C = 20		Moderate	Waitlist	Coping with the chronic condition in daily life	NA	MM + EM + RM	Individual	Education	NA	Online
Berrien et al. [46]	USA		HIV	N = 3 / I = 20 / C = 17		Moderate	Usual care	Adherence / Disease knowledge	NA	MM	Individual	Education	Nurse	Home
Betz et al. [47]	USA		Spina bifida	N = 65 / I = 31 / C = 34		Low	Usual care	Psychological outcomes	NA	MM + RM	Group	Goal-setting skills	NA	Clinic
Bignall et al. [19]	USA		Asthma	N = 30 / I = 14 / C = 16		Moderate	Usual care	Anxiety / Quality of life / Symptoms	NA	MM + EM	Group	Education / Relaxation training	Researchers	School
Breakey et al. [77]	Canada		Hemophilia	N = 29 / I = 16 / C = 13		Moderate	Usual care	Coping with the chronic condition in daily life / Disease knowledge / Quality of life	NA	MM + EM + RM	Individual	Education / Peer-support / Relaxation training / Telemedicine	Researchers	Online
Butz et al. [48]	USA		Asthma	N = 200 / I = 112 / C = 98		Moderate	Usual care	Coping with the chronic condition in daily life / Disease knowledge / Quality of life	NA	MM	Group	Education	Asthma educator	School
Canino et al. [20]	USA		Asthma	N = 221 / I = 110 / C = 111		High	Usual care	Adherence / School attendance / Symptoms	NA	MM	Individual	Education / Family therapy	Asthma counselor	Home

Study	Country	Condition	N	Quality	Control	Outcomes		MM/RM/EM	Format	Components	Physicians	Setting
Castensoe-Seidenfaden et al. [21]	Denmark	Diabetes type 1	N = 151; I = 76; C = 75	High	Usual care	Coping with the chronic condition in daily life; Symptoms	NA	MM + RM	Individual	Education; Peer-support; Self-monitoring	Nurse; Dietician	Online
Chiang et al. [49]	Taiwan	Asthma	N = 48; I = 22; C = 26	Moderate	Another specific intervention	Anxiety; Quality of life; Symptoms	NA	MM	Individual	Education; Relaxation training; Self-monitoring	Nurse (under-graduate degree)	Home; Clinic
Christian et al. [50]	USA	Cystic fibrosis	N = 116; I = 58; C = 58	High	Usual care	Quality of life; Symptoms	NA	RM	Individual; Group	Education; Peer-support; Problem-solving skills	NA	Home; Clinic
Connelly et al. [51]	USA	Migraine headache	N = 31; I = 14; C = 17	High	Waitlist	Symptoms	NA	MM + EM	Individual	Cognitive restructuring; Education; Relaxation training	NA	Home
Davis et al. [52]	USA	Cystic fibrosis	N = 47; I = 25; C = 22	High	Waitlist	Coping with the chronic condition in daily life; Disease knowledge	NA	MM + RM + EM	Individual	Education	NA	Home
Downs et al. [53]	Australia	Cystic fibrosis	N = 43; I = 18; C = 25	Moderate	Not clear	Adherence; Disease knowledge	CSL	MM	Individual	Decision-making skills; Education; Problem-solving skills	Healthcare professional	Clinic
Franklin et al. [54]	UK	Diabetes	N = 90; I1 = 32; I2 = 31; C = 27	Moderate	Another specific intervention	Adherence; Coping with the chronic condition in daily life; Disease knowledge; Symptoms	CSL	MM	Individual	Goal-setting skills; Telemedicine	Diabetes healthcare team	Clinic

(continued)

Table 4.2 (continued)

Background		Participants		Study characteristics			Components of self-management interventions					
Studies	Country	Chronic condition	N	Methodological Quality[a]	Control	Outcome measure	Theoretical base (Yes)[b]	Domain of self-management[c]	Formats	Elements	Interventionists	Setting
Freedenberg et al. [23]	USA	Congenital heart disease	N = 46	Low	Another specific intervention	Coping with the chronic condition in daily life	CBT	MM + EM	Group	Cognitive restructuring	NA	Clinic
			I = 26			Anxiety				Discussion		
			C = 20			Depression				Relaxation training		
Gross et al. [24]	Germany	Chronic abdominal pain	N = 29	High	Waitlist	Quality of life	NA	MM + EM	Group	Cognitive restructuring	Psychologist	NA
			I = 15			Symptoms				Education		
			C = 14							Relaxation training		
Haas et al. [25]	USA	Celiac disease	N = 61	Moderate	Usual care	Adherence	NA	MM	Individual	Education	Researcher Dietician	Online
			I = 31			Quality of life						
			C = 30			Symptoms						
Henkemans et al. [26]	The Netherlands	Diabetes type 1	N = 27	Moderate	Usual care	Coping with the chronic condition in daily life	Self-determination theory	MM	individual	Education	NA	Clinic (outpatient)
			I = 16			Disease knowledge						
			C = 11									
Hickman et al. [27]	USA	Migraine headache	N = 36	Moderate	Another specific intervention	Anxiety	CBT	MM + EM	NA	Education	Nurse (RN)	Clinic (outpatient)
			I = 18			Depression				Goal-setting skills		
			C = 18							Problem-solving skills		

Hommel et al. [28]	USA	Inflammatory bowel disease	N = 41 I = 20 C = 21	Moderate	Usual care	Adherence Coping with the chronic condition in daily life Quality of life	NA	MM + EM	Group	Discussion Education Goal-setting skills Problem-solving skills	Psychologist	Clinic (outpatient)
Huss et al. [55]	USA	Asthma	N = 101 I = 56 C = 45	Moderate	Usual care	Disease knowledge	NA	MM	Individual	Education	NA	Home
Jan et al. [56]	Taiwan	Asthma	N = 164 I = 88 C = 76	Moderate	Another specific intervention	Symptoms	NA	MM	Individual	Education Self-monitoring	NA	Clinic (outpatient)
Johnson et al. [29]	USA	Asthma	N = 89 I = 46 C = 43	Moderate	Usual care	Adherence Coping with the chronic condition in daily life Quality of life Symptoms	NA	MM	Individual	Self-monitoring	NA	Online
Jones et al. [57]	USA	Cancer	N = 65 I = 35 C = 30	Moderate	Another specific intervention	Coping with the chronic condition in daily life Disease knowledge	NA	MM + RM	Individual	Education	Healthcare professional	Home
Joseph et al. [58]	USA	Asthma	N = 314 I = 162 C = 152	Moderate	Another specific intervention	Quality of life School attendance Symptoms	Trans-theoretical/health belief model	MM	Individual	Education	NA	School
Kashikar-Zuck et al. [84], Kashikar-Zuck et al. [59]	USA	Juvenile fibro-myalgia	N = 114 I = 57 C = 57	High	Another specific intervention	Depression Symptoms	CBT	MM	Individual	Cognitive restructuring Education Problem-solving skills Relaxation training	Psychologist	Clinic

(continued)

Table 4.2 (continued)

Background			Participants		Study characteristics			Components of self-management interventions					
Studies	Country	Chronic condition	N	Methodological Quality[a]	Control	Outcome measure	Theoretical base (Yes)[b]	Domain of self-management[c]	Formats	Elements	Interventionists	Setting
Kato et al. [60]	USA	Cancer	N = 371 I = 195 C = 176	High	Another specific intervention	Adherence Coping with the chronic condition in daily life Disease knowledge Psychological outcomes Quality of life	CSL	MM	Individual	Education	NA	NA
Kazeminezhad et al. [30]	Iran	Diabetes type 1	N = 50 I = 25 C = 25	Moderate	Not clear	Symptoms	NA	MM	Group	Education	NA	NA
Koontz et al. [61]	USA	Sickle cell disease	N = 24 I = 10 C = 14	Low	Another specific intervention	Disease knowledge School attendance	NA	MM + RM	Group	Education Peer-support	Teachers	School
Korterink et al. [31]	The Netherlands	Inflammatory bowel disease	N = 69 I = 35 C = 34	high	Usual care	Quality of life School attendance Symptoms	NA	MM RM	Group	Relaxation training	NA	Clinic + Home
Krishna et al. [62]	USA	Asthma	N = 228 I = 107 C = 121	Moderate	Another specific intervention	Disease knowledge School attendance Symptoms	NA	MM	Individual	Decision-making skills Education Social skills	Multidisciplinary team	Clinic
Kumar et al. [63]	USA	Diabetes	N = 40 I = 19 C = 21	Moderate	Another specific intervention	Symptoms	NA	MM	Individual	Self-monitoring	NA	Online

Study	Country	Condition	N	Risk	Comparator	Outcomes	Theory	Mode	Format	Components	Provider	Setting
Laffel et al. [64]	USA	Diabetes	N = 100 I = 50 C = 50	Moderate	Usual care	Quality of life Symptoms	NA	MM	Individual	Family therapy Education Goal-setting skills	Research assistant	Clinic
Law et al. [32]	USA	Migraine headache	N = 83 I = 44 C = 39	High	Usual care	Anxiety Depression Symptoms	CBT	MM	Individual	Education Goal-setting Relaxation training	Psychologist	Online
Levy et al. [33]	USA	Inflammatory bowel disease	N = 185 I = 91 C = 94	Moderate	Another specific intervention	Coping with the chronic condition in daily life Psychological outcomes Symptoms Quality of life	SLT CBT	MM + EM	Individual	Cognitive restructuring Education Relaxation training	Therapist	Outpatient clinic
Mackie et al. [34]	Canada	Congenital heart disease	N = 121 I = 58 C = 63	Low	Usual care	Coping with the chronic condition in daily life Disease knowledge	NA	MM	Individual	Communication skills Discussion Education Goal-setting skills	Nurses	Outpatient clinic
Mcpherson et al. [78]	UK	Asthma	N = 101 I = 51 C = 50	Moderate	Another specific intervention	Disease knowledge Symptoms	NA	MM	Individual	Education Problem-solving skills Self-monitoring	NA	Home
McKillop et al. [35]	Canada	Congenital heart disease	N = 36 I = 18 C = 18	Moderate	Usual care	Coping with the chronic condition in daily life Quality of life	NA	MM	Individual	Education	NA	Phone

(continued)

Table 4.2 (continued)

Background		Participants		Study characteristics			Components of self-management interventions					
Studies	Country	Chronic condition	N	Methodological Quality[a]	Control	Outcome measure	Theoretical base (Yes)[b]	Domain of self-management[c]	Formats	Elements	Interventionists	Setting
Moghanloo et al. [36]	Iran	Diabetes type 1	N = 34; I = 17; C = 17	Moderate	Waitlist	Depression; Quality of life	Acceptance and commitment theory	EM	Group	NA	Psychologist	Clinic
Mulvaney et al. [79]	USA	Diabetes type 1	N = 49; I = 31; C = 18	Moderate	Usual care	Adherence; Symptoms	CSL; Self-determination theory	MM	Individual	Peer-support; Problem-solving skills	NA	Online
Naar-King et al. [80]	USA	HIV	T = 76; I = 36; C = 40	High	Another intervention	Adherence; Symptoms	NA	MM	Individual	Education; Goal-setting skills; Telemedicine	NA	Home
Newcombe et al. [65]	Australia	Chronic respiratory Condition	N = 39; I = 19; C = 20	High	Waitlist	Coping with the chronic condition in daily life; Depression	NA	MM	Individual; Group (online)	Education; Peer-support; Self-monitoring	NA	Online
Ng et al. [66]	China	Asthma	N = 37; I = 20; C = 17	Moderate	Waitlist	Quality of life; Symptoms	NA	MM + RM + EM	Group	Education; Family therapy	NA	Clinic
Nunn et al. [83]	Australia	Diabetes type 1	N = 139; I = 60; C = 63	Moderate	Usual Care	Disease knowledge	NA	MM	Individual	Education; Self-monitoring; Telemedicine	NA	Home
Palermo et al. [37, 67]; Fales et al. [22]	USA	Chronic pain	N = 48; I = 26; C = 22	High	Waitlist	Anxiety; Depression; Symptoms	CBT, CSL	MM	Individual	Cognitive restructuring; Education; Relaxation training	Psychologist	Online

Pulgaron et al. [68]	USA	Asthma	N = 41 I = 20 C = 21	Moderate	Usual care	Coping with the chronic condition in daily life Disease knowledge	NA	MM	Group	Education Peer-support Problem-solving skills	Psychologist (under-graduate degree)	Camp
Rapoff et al. [38]	USA	Migraine headache	N = 35 I = 18 C = 17	Low	Another specific intervention	Quality of life Symptoms	CBT	MM + EM	Individual	Education Problem-solving skills Relaxation training	Self-guided	CD-ROM
Rhee et al. [69]	USA	Asthma	N = 91 I = 46 C = 45	Moderate	Another specific intervention	Quality of life Symptoms	NA	MM + RM	Group	Discussion Education Peer-support Telemedicine	NA	Camp
Rostami et al. [39]	Iran	Diabetes type 1	N = 74 I = 37 C = 37	High	Waitlist	Depression Symptoms	NA	MM + EM	Group	Cognitive restructuring Discussion Education	Researcher	NA
Schatz et al. [40]	USA	Sickle cell disease	N = 46 I = 23 C = 23	Moderate	Waitlist	Coping with the chronic condition in daily life	CBT	MM	Group + individual	Cognitive restructuring Discussion Education Self-monitoring	Pediatric and psychiatric nurse	Clinic (outpatient) Telephone
Scholten et al. [70]	Netherlands	Chronic condition	N = 194 I1 = 71 I2 = 49 C = 74	Moderate	Waitlist	Psychological outcomes	NA	MM + EM + RM	Group	Cognitive restructuring Education Family therapy Relaxation techniques Social skills	Psychologist	Clinic School

(continued)

Table 4.2 (continued)

	Background	Participants			Study characteristics			Components of self-management interventions					
Studies	Country	Chronic condition	N	Methodological Quality[a]	Control	Outcome measure	Theoretical base (Yes)[b]	Domain of self-management[c]	Formats	Elements	Interventionists	Setting
Shames et al. [71]	USA	Asthma	N = 119 I = 59 C = 60	Moderate	Usual care	Disease knowledge Symptoms	NA	MM	Individual	Education Telemedicine	Case manager Clinician Nurse	Clinic Home
Staab et al. [72]	Germany	Atopic dermatitis	N = 823 I = 446 C = 377	Moderate	Another specific intervention	Symptoms	NA	MM + EM	Group	Education Peer-support Relaxation training	Dermatologist Pediatrician Psychologist Dieticians	Clinic
Stapersma et al. [41]	The Netherlands	Inflammatory bowel disease	N = 70 I = 37 C = 33	High	Usual care	Anxiety Depression Quality of life	CBT	MM + RM + EM	Group	Cognitive restructuring Education Social skills training	Therapist	Clinic (outpatient) Telephone
Stinson et al. [73]	Canada	Juvenile idiopathic arthritis	N = 46 I = 22 C = 24	High	Another specific intervention	Adherence Coping with the chronic condition in daily life Disease knowledge Psychological outcomes Quality of life Symptoms	NA	MM + RM + EM	Individual	Education Telemedicine	Psychologist (under-graduate degree)	Online
Stulemeijer et al. [74]	Netherlands	Chronic fatigue syndrome	N = 71 I = 36 C = 35	High	Waiting list	School attendance Symptoms	CBT	MM + RM + EM	Individual	Cognitive restructuring Education	Psychologist	Clinic
van Dijk-Lokkart et al. [42]	The Netherlands	Cancer	N = 68 I = 30 C = 38	Low	Usual care	Quality of life Symptoms	NA	MM + RM + EM	individual	Cognitive restructuring Education Relaxation training Social skills	Physiotherapist	Outpatient clinic

Study	Country	Condition	N	Quality	Control	Outcomes	Theory	MM	Format	Components	Provider	Setting
Velsor-Friedrich et al. [75]	USA	Asthma	N = 52 I = 28 C = 24	Low	Usual care	Symptoms	Orem's self-care deficit theory of nursing	MM + RM	Individual Group	Education Peer-support	Nurse practitioner	School
Walders et al. [81]	USA	Asthma	N = 175 I = 89 C = 86	Moderate	Usual care	Symptoms Quality of life	NA	MM	Individual	Education Problem-solving skills Telemedicine	Nurse Asthma social worker Psychologist	Clinic
Wei et al. [43]	UK	Diabetes type 1	N = 85 I = 43 C = 42	Low	Another specific intervention	Coping with the chronic condition in daily life Quality of life	CBT	MM + EM	Group	Cognitive restructuring Problem-solving sills Relaxation training Social skills	Psychologist	Home Clinic (outpatient)
Wiecha et al. [82]	USA	Asthma	N = 58 I = 37 C = 20	Low	Usual care	Adherence Symptoms	SCL	MM	Individual	Discussion Education Peer-support Self-monitoring	Physician Research assistant	Home
Wysocki et al. [76]	USA	Diabetes	N = 104 I = 28 C1 = 31 C2 = 26	Moderate	Another specific intervention Usual care	Adherence Symptoms	NA	MM + RM	Individual	Cognitive restructuring Communication skills Education Family therapy Problem-solving skills	Psychologist	Clinic

[a] Assessed using the methodology checklists of the Scottish Intercollegiate Guidelines Network (SIGN) for randomized controlled trials

[b] NA not available, CSL cognitive social learning theory, CBT cognitive behavioral theory

[c] MM medical management, EM emotional management, RM role management (according Lorig and Holman [141])

self-management is conceptualized differently in studies, resulting in a diversity of components and content of SMI, and a variety of outcome measurements used in the evaluation studies. In order to improve the (insights in) effectiveness of SMI, it is recommended to further standardize the development and evaluation of self-management interventions [6, 86, 87].

Most SMI were focused on the reduction of physical symptoms (52%), improving quality of life (30%), increasing disease knowledge (29%), or improving coping with the chronic condition in daily life (26%). Other SMI were focused on reducing depressive feelings (15%), or anxiety (11%) or non-adherence (14%), and on improving school attendance (8%). The evaluation studies published between 2016 and 2020 were mainly focused on psychological outcomes such as anxiety and depression, which points to a shift toward a broader operationalization of SMI, i.e., paying more attention to the emotional domain. This shift is important, because identifying and paying attention to adolescents' lived experiences and needs in the areas of emotional well-being and social participation during adolescence is essential for them to achieve their full potential and a satisfying adult life [88]. Although school attendance is considered as an important outcome of self-management support, less attention is paid to this outcome measure in evaluation studies [86, 89, 90].

4.3.3   General Effects of Self-Management Interventions

Thirty-four SMI were focused on the reduction of physical symptoms. Of these, more than half was either significantly effective (21%) or showed a positive trend in favor of the intervention group (44%). For those aimed at improving adherence ($n = 9$) these percentages were both 44.1%, and for those trying to increase disease knowledge ($n = 19$), these percentages were 53% and 37%, respectively. These findings are in line with those of previous studies, showing possible evidence for effectiveness of SMI on disease knowledge of youth with spina bifida, arthritis, asthma, or diabetes [86, 91–94] and for effectiveness of pediatric SMI on adherence [91, 95, 96], and symptom reduction [93, 94, 96, 97].

SMI also seem useful to improve HRQoL. Of the interventions that aimed to do so, 20% showed a significant positive effect and 50% showed a positive trend in the intervention group. Ten SMI were focused on reduction of depressive feelings. Of these, 30% was significantly effective and 30% showed a positive trend in favor of the intervention group. For those SMI aimed at coping with the chronic condition ($n = 17$) no clear effects were found: Only two studies (12%) showed a significant positive effect and only 41% showed a trend in favor of the intervention group. Finally, SMI that were focused on reducing anxiety, do not seem effective at all. Four out of seven (57%) of these even showed a positive trend in favor of the control group.

Conflicting evidence for effectiveness of SMI on patient-reported outcomes such as HRQoL have been reported in previous reviews [87, 97]. Although findings in this review have to be interpreted with caution, overall it seems that SMI do have positive effects on different outcomes. In the next paragraph we will explore further what elements in SMI may help or not.

4.3.4   Promising Intervention Components

An overview of promising interventions components per outcome measure category is presented in Table 4.3.

4.3.4.1 Outcomes of Self-Management Domains as Intervention Components

The fact that self-management is more than medical management is repeatedly emphasized in the self-management literature. Yet, a focus on the medical management domain seemed to be a promising component of SMI for a wide array of outcome categories, i.e., HRQoL, coping with the chronic condition in daily life, anxiety, depressive feelings, adherence, and disease knowledge. Perhaps a better understanding of the chronic condition and its treatment, helps to integrate these in daily life and could make the young people more confident in handling their situation. The different self-management domains are interrelated. As such, a focus on the medical domain may positively affect other (nonmedical) outcomes as well. An important addition is that no evidence was found that SMI focused on medical management could lead to reduced physical symptoms. To reduce symptoms, it seems to be important to pay attention to the emotional side of having a chronic condition as well. However, the results also suggest that the combination of emotional and medical domains should be avoided if the aim is to reduce anxiety or depressive feelings. No evidence was found for SMI targeting the role and emotional domains alone or the domains in other combinations, possibly due to the small number of SMI employing such approaches. Only recently, SMI seemed to tread the role and emotional domains and future research might shed some light on the effects thereof.

4.3.4.2 Professionals Involved as Intervention Components

SMI that were provided monodisciplinary (i.e., delivered by one type of healthcare professional) seemed to be promising in terms of reduced symptoms, increased disease knowledge, increased adherence, improved ability to deal with the chronic condition in daily life and reduced anxiety and depressive feelings of young people. Evidence for multidisciplinary provided SMI was only found for disease knowledge. This finding is somewhat unexpected, since the combination of different kinds of expertise of healthcare professionals was expected to result in an accumulation of knowledge and skills that could improve SMI effectiveness. Also, one could argue that, in order to cover all domains of self-management, different kinds of expertise are needed (e.g., expertise of a nurse, a psychologist, and an occupational therapist). However, most included SMI focused on a single self-management domain, thus the effects of multidisciplinary SMI are not clear. Also, the single focus and involvement of one discipline may lead to more specific and explicit intervention aims, benefitting (research into) effectiveness of SMI.

Most interventions were delivered by psychologists and such SMI seem to be promising in reducing physical symptoms, improving disease knowledge, dealing with the chronic condition, reducing anxiety and depressive feelings and fostering

Table 4.3 Effective intervention components per outcome measure[a]

Outcomes	Symptom reduction	Disease knowledge	Adherence	Dealing with the chronic condition in daily life	Anxiety	Depressive feelings	School attendance	Quality of life
SMI component								
SM domain								
MM	-/+	+	+	+	+	+	-/+	+
MM + EM	+			-/+	-	-		+
MM + EM + RM	+	+		+			-/+	-/+
EM						-/+		-/+
EM + RM			-/+				-/+	
RM	-/+							-/+
RM + MM	-/+	-/+	-/+	-/+			-/+	-/+
Discipline (number of studies)[a]								
Monodisciplinary	+	+	+	+	+	+	-/+	-/+
Multidisciplinary	-/+	+	-/+	-/+			-/+	
Format (number of studies)[a]								
Individual	-/+	+	+	+	+	-/+	-/+	-/+
Group	+	-/+		-/+	-	-/+	-/+	+
Individual and group				-/+		-/+		-/+
Interventionists (number of studies)[a]								
Psychologist	+	+	-/+	+	+	+	-/+	+
Nurse	-/+	-/+	-/+		-/+	-/+		-/+
Peers		-/+		-/+				-/+
Setting (number of studies)[a]								
Clinic	+	+	+	+	-/+	+	-/+	+

Home	-/+	+	+	+		-/+	-/+
School	+	-	-/+	-/+	-/+	-/+	+
Online	-	-/+			-/+		-/+
Home and clinic	+	-/+	-/+	-/+			+
Camp	-/+	-/+	-/+				

a+ = we found evidence for effectiveness of the intervention component on the specific outcome measure, − = we found evidence for this intervention component not to be effective on the specific outcome measure, −/+ = no evidence was found

HRQoL. This is not surprising, since SMI focused on these outcomes usually aimed to intervene on cognitions, coping and behavior, and this is the expertise area of a psychologist. For other professionals, effects were unclear since the number of studies with SMI delivered by non-psychologists was very low.

4.3.4.3 Formats as Intervention Components

Most SMI were delivered individually compared to those in groups (or a combination of both). Such SMI seemed to be promising in improving young people's ability to deal with their chronic condition, their disease knowledge and adherence and in reducing their anxiety. Group-based SMI were found to be promising in reducing symptoms and increasing HRQoL. However, if the aim is to reduce anxiety, group interventions should be avoided, since they do not seem to be effective in reducing anxiety. Perhaps this can be explained by sharing experiences during group sessions. The experience of one person with progressive symptoms of their chronic condition for instance, could make other group-members anxious about their own future. This is indeed mentioned as one of the possible negative effects of peer-support (also see Chap. 7). At the same time, peer-support is reported to decrease feelings of loneliness, improve social skills, increase social contacts, and improve positive attitudes toward having a chronic condition [98], which might explain the evidence we found for increased HRQoL.

4.3.4.4 Settings as Intervention Component

The clinic as setting seemed to be promising for almost all outcome categories, except for anxiety and school attendance. No effects for anxiety and school attendance were found for any of the settings. Interesting is that for HRQoL to improve, the home setting also seemed to be important, as it seemed promising both alone and in combination with the clinic setting. The combination home and clinic also seems good for reduction of symptoms. SMI delivered at home only furthermore showed promising effects for improving disease knowledge, adherence and dealing with the chronic conditions in daily life. Surprisingly, the last was also more achieved if the SMI was delivered online. Two components in combination with outcome categories were clearly not effective: interventions at school trying to improve disease knowledge and interventions online aiming to reduce symptoms. Overall, the clinic seems to be the most promising setting for SMI.

4.4   Key Recommendations for Practice

These recommendations are based on the results of our analysis. It is good to keep in mind that little is known about other elements than the ones mentioned and that we did not explore possible effects of the combination of elements.

Recommendations for Practice

- To reduce physical symptoms of young people with chronic conditions, use SMI with one or more of the following characteristics: SMI focusing on (a combination of) medical and role or medical, role and emotional management; delivered monodisciplinary and in a group; delivered by a psychologist in a clinic, at home, or a combination of both. It is not advisable to deliver such SMI online.
- To improve disease knowledge of young people with chronic conditions, use SMI with one or more of the following characteristics: focused on medical management alone or on all three self-management domains; can be delivered both mono- and multidisciplinary; targeted at individuals; can be delivered by psychologists at a clinic or at home. The school setting is not beneficial for such SMI.
- To improve adherence of young people with chronic conditions, use SMI with one or more of the following characteristics: focused on medical management; delivered monodisciplinary and individually in a clinic or at home.
- To improve the way young people cope with their chronic condition in daily life, use SMI with one or more of the following characteristics: focused on medical management alone or on all three self-management domains; delivered monodisciplinary, individually and by a psychologist at a clinic, at home or online.
- To reduce anxiety of young people with chronic conditions, use SMI with one or more of the following characteristics: focused on medical management; delivered monodisciplinary, individually, and by a psychologist. Do not use SMI focused on the combination of medical and emotional management and do not use group SMI.
- To reduce depressive feelings of young people with chronic conditions, use SMI with one or more of the following characteristics: focused on medical management, delivered monodisciplinary, by a psychologist and in a clinic. Not effective is the use of a SMI that focuses on both medical and emotional management.
- To improve health-related quality of life of young people with chronic conditions, use SMI with one or more of the following characteristics: focused on medical management alone or a combination of medical and emotional management; delivered in a group and by a psychologist; delivered at a clinic, at school or both at a clinic and at home.

4.5   Conclusion

Self-management support is important for young people growing with chronic conditions to help them deal with their condition in daily life, since they have to face the normal tasks of development (e.g., acquiring autonomy) and have to engage in lifelong medical management of their condition. In the last five years, there has been a shift in the focus of self-management support from mere medical management to a broader operationalization of SMI, including emotional and social aspects of dealing with a chronic condition. Not much can be said about promising intervention components of SMI, since a lot is unclear and for most of the combinations of components and outcome categories, no evidence was found due to the small number of studies that included these combinations. Still, available evidence showed that, depending on the selected outcome (i.e., aims of the SMI), promising intervention elements can be: a focus on medical management, monodisciplinary delivery, delivered by a psychologist, individual or group (they are complementary to each other) and delivered in a clinic. However, this is not to say that other intervention components are not effective, since no evidence found does not necessarily mean that those other components are not effective. Finally, relatively little is known about components that positively affect school attendance, depressive feelings, anxiety, and adherence.

4.6 Appendix: Evidence Profile

Outcome (No of studies)	Quality assessment					Number of patients		Quality of the evidence
	Limitation in design[a]	Inconsistency[b]	Indirectness[c]	Imprecision[d]	Publication bias[e]	C[f]	I[g]	
Symptoms (34)	No serious limitation	Very serious inconsistency	No serious indirectness	Serious imprecision	Unlikely	1480	1433	Very low
Disease knowledge (19)	No serious limitation	Serious inconsistency	No serious indirectness	No serious imprecision	Unlikely	839	788	Moderate
Adherence (9)	No serious limitation	Serious inconsistency	No serious indirectness	Serious imprecision	Unlikely	370	320	Low
Dealing with chronic condition in daily life (17)	No serious limitation	Very serious inconsistency	No serious indirectness	No serious limitation	Unlikely	664	616	Low
Anxiety (7)	No serious limitation	Serious inconsistency	No serious indirectness	Very serious imprecision	Unlikely	273	264	Very low
Depression (10)	No serious limitation	Serious inconsistency	No serious indirectness	No serious limitation	Unlikely	383	370	Moderate
School attendance (5)	No serious limitation	Serious inconsistency	Serious indirectness	Serious imprecision	Unlikely	285	305	Very low
Quality of life (20)	No serious limitation	Serious inconsistency	No serious indirectness	No serious limitation	Unlikely	926	875	Moderate

[a]Assessment of methodological quality
[b]Heterogeneity or variability in results across studies
[c]Indirect comparison of interventions within the studies
[d]Wide confidence intervals around the estimate of the effect
[e]Underestimating or overestimating of the effect due to the selective publication of studies
[f]Number of patients that participated in the control condition
[g]Number of patients that participated in the intervention condition

References

1. Harvey PW, Petkov JN, Misan G, Fuller J, Battersby MW, Cayetano TN, et al. Self-management support and training for patients with chronic and complex conditions improves health-related behaviour and health outcomes. Aust Health Rev. 2008;32(2):330–8. https://doi.org/10.1071/ah080330.
2. Wagner EH. Chronic disease management: what will it take to improve care for chronic illness? Eff Clin Pract. 1998;1(1):2–4.
3. Trappenburg J, Jonkman N, Jaarsma T, van Os-Medendorp H, Kort H, de Wit N, et al. Self-management: one size does not fit all. Patient Educ Couns. 2013;92(1):134–7. https://doi.org/10.1016/j.pec.2013.02.009.
4. Lindsay S, Kingsnorth S, McDougall C, Keating H. A systematic review of self-management interventions for children and youth with physical disabilities. Disabil Rehabil. 2014;36(4):276–88. https://doi.org/10.3109/09638288.2013.785605.
5. Kirk S, Beatty S, Callery P, Gellatly J, Milnes L, Pryjmachuk S. The effectiveness of self-care support interventions for children and young people with long-term conditions: a systematic review. Child Care Health Dev. 2012;39(3):305–24. https://doi.org/10.1111/j.1365-2214.2012.01395.x.
6. Nolte E, McKee M. Caring for people with chronic conditions: an introduction. In: Nolte E, McKee M, editors. Caring for people with chronic conditions. A health system perspective. Berkshire: Open University Press; 2008. https://doi.org/10.1055/s-0029-1239177.
7. Wagner EH, Austin BT, Davis C, Hindmarsh M, Schaefer J, Bonomi A. Improving chronic illness care: translating evidence into action. Health Aff. 2001;20(6):64–78. https://doi.org/10.1377/hlthaff.20.6.64.
8. Saxby N, Beggs S, Battersby M, Lawn S. What are the components of effective chronic condition self-management education interventions for children with asthma, cystic fibrosis, and diabetes? A systematic review. Patient Educ Couns. 2019;102(4):607–22. https://doi.org/10.1016/j.pec.2018.11.001.
9. Perrin JM, MacLean WE Jr, Gortmaker SL, Asher KN. Improving the psychological status of children with asthma: a randomized controlled trial. J Dev Behav Pediatr. 1992;13(4):241–7. https://doi.org/10.1097/00004703-199208000-00001.
10. Stein RE, Jessop DJ. What diagnosis does not tell: the case for a noncategorical approach to chronic illness in childhood. Soc Sci Med. 1989;29(6):769–78. https://doi.org/10.1016/0277-9536(89)90157-3.
11. Sawyer SM, Drew S, Yeo MS, Britto MT. Adolescents with a chronic condition: challenges living, challenges treating. Lancet. 2007;369(9571):1481–9.12. https://doi.org/10.1016/S0140-6736(07)60370-5.
12. Bal MI, Sattoe JN, Roelofs PD, Bal R, van Staa A, Miedema HS. Exploring effectiveness and effective components of self-management interventions for young people with chronic physical conditions: a systematic review. Patient Educ Couns. 2016;99(8):1293–309. https://doi.org/10.1016/j.pec.2016.02.012.
13. Scottish Intercollegiate Guidelines Network. Critical appraisal: notes and checklists. 2013. http://www.sign.ac.uk/methodology/checklists.html#.
14. Lorig KR, Holman H. Self-management education: history, definition, outcomes, and mechanisms. Ann Behav Med. 2003;26(1):1–7. https://doi.org/10.1207/S15324796ABM2601_01.
15. Higgins JPT, Green S, editors. Cochrane handbook for systematic reviews of interventions version 5.1.0 [updated March 2011]. London: The Cochrane Collaboration; 2011. www.handbook.cochrane.org.
16. DerSimonian R, Laird N. Meta-analysis in clinical trials. Control Clin Trials. 1986;7:177–88. https://doi.org/10.1016/j.cct.2015.09.002.
17. Ammerlaan J, van Os-Medendorp H, de Boer-Nijhof N, Scholtus L, Kruize AA, van Pelt P, et al. Short term effectiveness and experiences of a peer guided web-based self-management intervention for young adults with juvenile idiopathic arthritis. Pediatr Rheumatol. 2017;15:75. https://doi.org/10.1186/s12969-017-0201-1.

18. Beheshtipoor N, Sh G, Edraki M, Karimi M, Haghpanah S. The effects of computer-based educational games on self-efficacy of 8-12 children with hemophilia. Iran J Blood Cancer. 2015;7(3):157–62.
19. Bignall WJR, Luberto CM, Cornette AF, Haj-Hamed M, Cotton S. Breathing retraining for African-American adolescents with asthma: a pilot study of a school-based randomized controlled trial. J Asthma. 2015;52(9):889–96. https://doi.org/10.3109/02770903.2015.1033724.
20. Canino G, Vila D, Normand SLT, Acosta-Pérez E. Reducing asthma health disparities in poor Puerto Rican children: the effectiveness of a culturally tailored family intervention. Amsterdam: Elsevier; 2008. https://doi.org/10.1016/j.jaci.2007.10.022.
21. Castensoe-Seidenfaden P, Husted GR, Jensen AK, Hommel E, Olsen B, Pedersen-Bjergaard U, et al. Testing a smartphone app (young with diabetes) to improve self-management of diabetes over 12 months: randomized controlled trial. JMIR Mhealth Uhealth. 2018;6(6):e141. https://doi.org/10.2196/mhealth.9487.
22. Fales J, Palermo TM, Law EF, Wilson AC. Sleep outcomes in youth with chronic pain participating in a randomized controlled trial of online cognitive-behavioral therapy for pain management. Behav Sleep Med. 2015;13(2):107–23. https://doi.org/10.1080/1540200 2.2013.845779.
23. Freedenberg VA, Hinds PS, Friedmann E. Mindfulness-based stress reduction and group support decrease stress in adolescents with cardiac diagnoses: a randomized two-group study. Pediatr Cardiol. 2017;38(7):1415–25. https://doi.org/10.1007/s00246-017-1679-5.
24. Groß M, Warschburger P. Evaluation of a cognitive–behavioral pain management program for children with chronic abdominal pain: a randomized controlled study. Int J Behav Med. 2013;20(3):434–43. https://doi.org/10.1007/s12529-012-9228-3.
25. Haas K, Martin A, Park KJ. Text message intervention (TEACH) improves quality of life and patient activation in celiac disease: a randomized clinical trial. J Pediatr. 2017;185:62–7. https://doi.org/10.1016/j.jpeds.2017.02.062.
26. Henkemans OAB, Bierman BPB, Janssen J, Looije R, Neerincx MA, van Dooren MMM, et al. Design and evaluation of a personal robot playing a self-management education game with children with diabetes type 1. Int J Hum Comput Stud. 2017;106:63–76. https://doi.org/10.1016/j.ijhcs.2017.06.001.
27. Hickman C, Jacobson D, Melnyk BM. Randomized controlled trial of the acceptability, feasibility, and preliminary effects of a cognitive behavioral skills building intervention in adolescents with chronic daily headaches: a pilot study. J Pediatr Health Care. 2015;29(1):5–16. https://doi.org/10.1016/j.pedhc.2014.05.001.
28. Hommel KA, Hente EA, Odell S, Herzer M. Evaluation of a group-based behavioral intervention to promote adherence in adolescents with inflammatory bowel disease. Eur J Gastroenterol Hepatol. 2012;24(1):64–9. https://doi.org/10.1097/MEG.0b013e32834d09f1.
29. Johnson KB, Patterson BL, Yun-Xian H, Qingxia C, Hui N, Davison CL, et al. The feasibility of text reminders to improve medication adherence in adolescents with asthma. J Am Med Inform Assoc. 2016;23(3):449–55. https://doi.org/10.1093/jamia/ocv158.
30. Kazeminezhad B, Taghinejad H, Borji M, Tarjoman A. The effect of self-care on glycated hemoglobin and fasting blood sugar levels on adolescents with diabetes. J Compr Pediatr. 2018;9(2):e62661. https://doi.org/10.5812/compreped.62661.
31. Korterink JJ, Ockeloen LE, Hilbink M, Benninga MA, Deckers-Kocken JM. Yoga therapy for abdominal pain-related functional gastrointestinal disorders in children: a randomized controlled trial. J Pediatr Gastroenterol Nutr. 2016;63(5):481–7. https://doi.org/10.1097/MPG.0000000000001230.
32. Law EF, Beals-Erickson SE, Noel M, Claar R, Palermo TM. Pilot randomized controlled trial of internet-delivered cognitive-behavioral treatment for pediatric headache. Headache. 2015;55(10):1410–25. https://doi.org/10.1111/head.12635.
33. Levy RL, Van Tilburg MA, Langer SL, Romano JM, Walker LS, Mancl LA, et al. Effects of a cognitive behavioral therapy intervention trial to improve disease outcomes in children with inflammatory bowel disease. Inflamm Bowel Dis. 2016;22(9):2134–48. https://doi.org/10.1097/MIB.0000000000000881.

34. Mackie AS, Rempel GR, Kovacs AH, Kaufman M, Rankin KN, Jelen A, et al. Transition intervention for adolescents with congenital heart disease. J Am Coll Cardiol. 2018;71(16):1768–77. https://doi.org/10.1016/j.jacc.2018.02.043.

35. McKillop A, Grace SL, Ghisi GLM, Allison KR, Banks L, Kovacs AH, et al. Adapted motivational interviewing to promote exercise in adolescents with congenital heart disease: a pilot trial. Pediatr Phys Ther. 2018;30(4):326–34. https://doi.org/10.1097/PEP.0000000000000534.

36. Moghanloo VA, Moghanloo RA, Moazezi M. Effectiveness of acceptance and commitment therapy for depression, psychological well-being and feeling of guilt in 7-15 years old diabetic children. Iran J Pediatr. 2015;25(4):1–6. https://doi.org/10.5812/ijp.2436.

37. Palermo TM, Law EF, Fales J, Bromberg MH, Jessen-Fiddick T, Tai G. Internet-delivered cognitive-behavioral treatment for adolescents with chronic pain and their parents: a randomized controlled multicenter trial. Pain. 2016;157(1):174–85. https://doi.org/10.1097/j.pain.0000000000000348.

38. Rapoff MA, Connelly M, Bickel JL, Powers SW, Hershey AD, Allen JR, et al. Headstrong intervention for pediatric migraine headache: a randomized clinical trial. J Headache Pain. 2014;15(1):1–10. https://doi.org/10.1186/1129-2377-15-12.

39. Rostami S, Naseri M, Dashtbozorgi B, Zarea K, Riaahi Qhahfarrokhi K, Haghighizadeh MH. Effects of group training on depression and anxiety among patients with type i diabetes: a randomized clinical trial. BMJ Open. 2016;4(5):1777–86. https://doi.org/10.22038/IJP.2016.6740.

40. Schatz J, Schlenz AM, McClellan CB, Puffer ES, Hardy S, Pfeiffer M, et al. Changes in coping, pain, and activity after cognitive-behavioral training: a randomized clinical trial for pediatric sickle cell disease using smartphones. Clin J Pain. 2015;31(6):536–47. https://doi.org/10.1097/AJP.0000000000000183.

41. Stapersma L, van den Brink G, van der Ende J, Szigethy EM, Beukers R, Korpershoek TA, et al. Effectiveness of disease-specific cognitive behavioral therapy on anxiety, depression, and quality of life in youth with inflammatory bowel disease: a randomized controlled trial. J Pediatr Psychol. 2018;43(9):967–80. https://doi.org/10.1093/jpepsy/jsy029.

42. van Dijk-Lokkart EM, Braam KI, van Dulmen-den Broeder E, Kaspers GJ, Takken T, Grootenhuis MA, et al. Effects of a combined physical and psychosocial intervention program for childhood cancer patients on quality of life and psychosocial functioning: results of the QLIM randomized clinical trial. Psychooncology. 2016;25(7):815–22. https://doi.org/10.1002/pon.4016.

43. Wei C, Allen RJ, Tallis PM, Ryan FJ, Hunt LP, Shield JP, et al. Cognitive behavioural therapy stabilises glycaemic control in adolescents with type 1 diabetes—outcomes from a randomised control trial. Pediatr Diabetes. 2018;19(1):106–13. https://doi.org/10.1111/pedi.12519.

44. Barakat LP, Schwartz LA, Salamon KS, Radcliffe J. A family-based randomized controlled trial of pain intervention for adolescents with sickle cell disease. J Pediatr Hematol Oncol. 2010;32(7):540–7. https://doi.org/10.1097/MPH.0b013e3181e793f9.

45. Beebe A, Gelfand EW, Bender B. A randomized trial to test the effectiveness of art therapy for children with asthma. J Allergy Clin Immunol. 2010;126(2):263–U14. https://doi.org/10.1016/j.jaci.2010.03.019.

46. Berrien VM, Salazar JC, Reynolds E, McKay K, Group HIVMAI. Adherence to antiretroviral therapy in HIV-infected pediatric patients improves with home-based intensive nursing intervention. AIDS Patient Care STDS. 2004;18(6):355–63. https://doi.org/10.1089/1087291041444078.

47. Betz CL, Smith K, Macias K. Testing the transition preparation training program: a randomized controlled trial. Int J Child Adolesc Health. 2011;3(4):595–607. https://doi.org/10.1186/s12877-018-0792-5.

48. Butz A, Pham L, Lewis L, Lewis C, Hill K, Walker J, et al. Rural children with asthma: impact of a parent and child asthma education program. J Asthma. 2005;42(10):813–21. https://doi.org/10.1080/02770900500369850.

49. Chiang LC, Ma WF, Huang JL, Tseng LF, Hsueh KC. Effect of relaxation-breathing training on anxiety and asthma signs/symptoms of children with moderate-to-severe asthma: a randomized controlled trial. Int J Nurs Stud. 2009;46(8):1061–70. https://doi.org/10.1016/j.ijnurstu.2009.01.013.
50. Christian BJ, D'Auria JP. Building life skills for children with cystic fibrosis: effectiveness of an intervention. Nurs Res. 2006;55(5):300–7. https://doi.org/10.1097/00006199-200609000-00002.
51. Connelly M, Rapoff MA, Thompson N, Connelly W. Headstrong: a pilot study of a CD-ROM intervention for recurrent pediatric headache. J Pediatr Psychol. 2006;31(7):737–47. https://doi.org/10.1093/jpepsy/jsj003.
52. Davis MA, Quittner AL, Stack CM, Yang MCK. Controlled evaluation of the STARBRIGHT CD-ROM program for children and adolescents with cystic fibrosis. J Pediatr Psychol. 2004;29(4):259–67. https://doi.org/10.1093/jpepsy/jsh026.
53. Downs JA, Roberts CM, Blackmore AM, Le Souef PN, Jenkins SC. Benefits of an education programme on the self-management of aerosol and airway clearance treatments for children with cystic fibrosis. Chron Respir Dis. 2006;3(1):19–27. https://doi.org/10.1191/1479972306cd100oa.
54. Franklin VL, Waller A, Pagliari C, Greene SA. A randomized controlled trial of Sweet Talk, a text-messaging system to support young people with diabetes. Diabet Med. 2006;23(12):1332–8. https://doi.org/10.1111/j.1464-5491.2006.01989.x.
55. Huss K, Winkelstein M, Nanda J, Naumann PL, Sloand ED, Huss RW. Computer game for inner-city children does not improve asthma outcomes. J Pediatr Healthcare. 2003;17(2):72–8. https://doi.org/10.1067/mph.2003.28.
56. Jan RL, Wang JY, Huang MC, Tseng SM, Su HJ, Liu LF. An internet-based interactive tele-monitoring system for improving childhood asthma outcomes in Taiwan. Telemed J E Health. 2007;13(3):257–68. https://doi.org/10.1089/tmj.2006.0053.
57. Jones JK, Kamani SA, Bush PJ, Hennessy KA, Marfatia A, Shad AT. Development and evaluation of an educational interactive CD-ROM for teens with cancer. Pediatr Blood Cancer. 2010;55(3):512–9. https://doi.org/10.1002/pbc.22608.
58. Joseph CL, Peterson E, Havstad S, Johnson CC, Hoerauf S, Stringer S, et al. A web-based, tailored asthma management program for urban African-American high school students. Am J Respir Crit Care Med. 2007;175(9):888–95. https://doi.org/10.1164/rccm.200608-1244OC.
59. Kashikar-Zuck S, Ting TV, Arnold LM, Bean J, Powers SW, Graham TB, et al. Cognitive behavioral therapy for the treatment of juvenile fibromyalgia: a multisite, single-blind, randomized, controlled clinical trial. Arthritis Rheum. 2012;64(1):297–305. https://doi.org/10.1002/art.30644.
60. Kato PM, Cole SW, Bradlyn AS, Pollock BH. A video game improves behavioral outcomes in adolescents and young adults with cancer: a randomized trial. Pediatrics. 2008;122(2):305–17. https://doi.org/10.1542/peds.2007-3134.
61. Koontz K, Short AD, Kalinyak K, Noll RB. A randomized, controlled pilot trial of a school intervention for children with sickle cell anemia. J Pediatr Psychol. 2004;29(1):7–17. https://doi.org/10.1093/jpepsy/jsh002.
62. Krishna S, Francisco BD, Balas EA, Konig P, Graff GR, Madsen RW, et al. Internet-enabled interactive multimedia asthma education program: a randomized trial. Pediatrics. 2003;111(3):503–10. https://doi.org/10.1542/peds.111.3.503.
63. Kumar VS, Wentzell KJ, Mikkelsen T, Pentland A, Laffel LM. The DAILY (Daily Automated Intensive Log for Youth) trial: a wireless, portable system to improve adherence and glycemic control in youth with diabetes. Diabetes Technol Ther. 2004;6(4):445–53. https://doi.org/10.1089/1520915041705893.
64. Laffel LM, Vangsness L, Connell A, Goebel-Fabbri A, Butler D, Anderson BJ. Impact of ambulatory, family-focused teamwork intervention on glycemic control in youth with type 1 diabetes. J Pediatr. 2003;142(4):409–16. https://doi.org/10.1067/mpd.2003.138.

65. Newcombe PA, Dunn TL, Casey LM, Sheffield JK, Petsky H, Anderson-James S, et al. Breathe easier online: evaluation of a randomized controlled pilot trial of an internet-based intervention to improve well-being in children and adolescents with a chronic respiratory condition. J Med Internet Res. 2012;14(1):115–26. https://doi.org/10.2196/jmir.1997.

66. Ng SM, Li AM, Lou VW, Tso IF, Wan PY, Chan DF. Incorporating family therapy into asthma group intervention: a randomized waitlist-controlled trial. Fam Process. 2008;47(1):115–30. https://doi.org/10.1111/j.1545-5300.2008.00242.x.

67. Palermo TM, Wilson AC, Peters M, Lewandowski A, Somhegyi H. Randomized controlled trial of an Internet-delivered family cognitive-behavioral therapy intervention for children and adolescents with chronic pain. Pain. 2009;146(1–2):205–13. https://doi.org/10.1016/j.pain.2009.07.034.

68. Pulgaron ER, Salamon KS, Patterson CA, Barakat LP. A problem-solving intervention for children with persistent asthma: a pilot of a randomized trial at a pediatric summer camp. J Asthma. 2010;47(9):1031–9. https://doi.org/10.1080/02770903.2010.514633.

69. Rhee H, Belyea MJ, Hunt JF, Brasch J. Effects of a peer-led asthma self-management program for adolescents. Arch Pediatr Adolesc Med. 2011;165(6):513–9. https://doi.org/10.1001/archpediatrics.2011.79.

70. Scholten L, Willemen AM, Grootenhuis MA, Maurice-Stam H, Schuengel C, Last BF. A cognitive behavioral based group intervention for children with a chronic illness and their parents: a multicentre randomized controlled trial. BMC Pediatr. 2011;11:1–8. https://doi.org/10.1186/1471-2431-11-65.

71. Shames RS, Sharek P, Mayer M, Robinson TN, Hoyte EG, Gonzalez-Hensley F, et al. Effectiveness of a multicomponent self-management program in at-risk, school-aged children with asthma. Ann Allergy Asthma Immunol. 2004;92(6):611–8. https://doi.org/10.1016/S1081-1206(10)61426-3.

72. Staab D, Diepgen TL, Fartasch M, Kupfer J, Lob-Corzilius T, Ring J, et al. Age related, structured educational programmes for the management of atopic dermatitis in children and adolescents: multicentre, randomised controlled trial. BMJ. 2006;332(7547):933–8. https://doi.org/10.1136/bmj.332.7547.933.

73. Stinson JN, McGrath PJ, Hodnett ED, Feldman BM, Duffy CM, Huber AM, et al. An internet-based self-management program with telephone support for adolescents with arthritis: a pilot randomized controlled trial. J Rheumatol. 2010;37(9):1944–52. https://doi.org/10.3899/jrheum.091327.

74. Stulemeijer M, De Jong LWAM, Fiselier TJW, Hoogveld SWB, Bleijenberg G. Cognitive behaviour therapy for adolescents with chronic fatigue syndrome: randomised controlled trial. Br Med J. 2005;330(7481):14–7. https://doi.org/10.1136/bmj.38301.587106.63.

75. Velsor-Friedrich B, Pigott T, Srof B. A practitioner-based asthma intervention program with African American inner-city school children. J Pediatr Healthcare. 2005;19(3):163–71. https://doi.org/10.1016/j.pedhc.2004.12.002.

76. Wysocki T, Harris MA, Buckloh LM, Mertlich D, Lochrie AS, Mauras N, et al. Randomized trial of behavioral family systems therapy for diabetes: maintenance of effects on diabetes outcomes in adolescents. Diabetes Care. 2007;30(3):555–60. https://doi.org/10.2337/dc06-1613.

77. Breakey VR, Ignas DM, Warias AV, White M, Blanchette VS, Stinson JN. A pilot randomized control trial to evaluate the feasibility of an Internet-based self-management and transitional care program for youth with haemophilia. Haemophilia. 2014;20(6):784–93. https://doi.org/10.1111/hae.12488.

78. McPherson AC, Glazebrook C, Forster D, James C, Smyth A. A randomized, controlled trial of an interactive educational computer package for children with asthma. Pediatrics. 2006;117(4):1046–54. https://doi.org/10.1542/peds.2005-0666.

79. Mulvaney SA, Rothman RL, Wallston KA, Lybarger C, Dietrich MS. An internet-based program to improve self-management in adolescents with type 1 diabetes. Diabetes Care. 2010;33(3):602–4. https://doi.org/10.2337/dc09-1881.

80. Naar-King S, Outlaw AY, Sarr M, Parsons JT, Belzer M, Macdonell K, et al. Motivational Enhancement System for Adherence (MESA): pilot randomized trial of a brief computer-delivered prevention intervention for youth initiating antiretroviral treatment. J Pediatr Psychol. 2013;38(6):638–48. https://doi.org/10.1093/jpepsy/jss132.

81. Walders N, Kercsmar C, Schluchter M, Redline S, Kirchner HL, Drotar D. An interdisciplinary intervention for undertreated pediatric asthma. Chest. 2006;129(2):292–9. https://doi.org/10.1378/chest.129.2.292.

82. Wiecha JM, Adams WG, Rybin D, Rizzodepaoli M, Keller J, Clay JM. Evaluation of a web-based asthma self-management system: a randomised controlled pilot trial. BMC Polm Med. 2015;15(1):7. https://doi.org/10.1186/s12890-015-0007-1.

83. Nunn E, King B, Smart C, Anderson D. A randomized controlled trial of telephone calls to young patients with poorly controlled type 1 diabetes. Pediatr Diabetes. 2006;7(5):254–9. https://doi.org/10.1111/j.1399-5448.2006.00200.x.

84. Kashikar-Zuck S, Swain NF, Jones BA, Graham TB. Efficacy of cognitive-behavioral intervention for juvenile primary fibromyalgia syndrome. J Rheumatol. 2005;32(8):1594–602. https://doi.org/10.1002/art.30644.

85. Al-sheyab N, Gallagher R, Crisp J, Shah S. Peer-led education for adolescents with asthma in Jordan: a cluster-randomized controlled trial. Pediatrics. 2012;129(1):e106–12. https://doi.org/10.1542/peds.2011-0346.

86. Gall C, Kingsnorth S, Healy H. Growing up ready: a shared management approach. Phys Occup Ther Pediatr. 2006;26:47–62. https://doi.org/10.1080/J006v26n04_04.

87. Nolte S, Osborne RH. A systematic review of outcomes of chronic disease self-management interventions. Qual Life Res. 2013;22:1805–16. https://doi.org/10.1007/s11136-012-0302-8.

88. Maslow GR, Haydon A, McRee AL, et al. Growing up with a chronic illness: social success, educational/vocational distress. J Adolesc Health. 2011;49:206–12. https://doi.org/10.1016/j.jadohealth.2010.12.001.

89. Lopez-Vargas P, Tong A, Crowe S, Alexander SI, Caldwell PHY, Campbell DE. Research priorities for childhood chronic conditions: a workshop report. Arch Dis Child. 2019;104:237–45. https://doi.org/10.1136/archdischild-2018-315628.

90. Maurice-Stam H, Nijhof SL, Monninkhof AS, Heymans HAS, Grootenhuis MA. Review about the impact of growing up with a chronic disease showed delays achieving psychosocial milestones. Acta Paediatr. 2019;00:1–13. https://doi.org/10.1111/apa.1491891.

91. Bravata DM, Gienger AL, Holty JE, Sundaram V, Khazeni N, Wise PH, McDonald KM, Owens DK. Quality improvement strategies for children with asthma: a systematic review. Arch Pediatr Adolesc Med. 2009;163:572–81. https://doi.org/10.1001/archpediatrics.2009.63.

92. Irwin CW. Young adults are worse off than adolescents. J Adolesc Health. 2010;46:405–6. https://doi.org/10.1016/j.jadohealth.2010.03.001.

93. DeShazo J, Harris L, Pratt W. Effective intervention or child's play? A review of video games for diabetes education. Diabetes Technol Ther. 2010;12:815–22. https://doi.org/10.1089/dia.2010.0030.

94. Russell-Minda E, Jutai J, Speechley M, Bradley K, Chudyk A, Petrella R. Health technologies for monitoring and managing diabetes: a systematic review. J Diabetes Sci Technol. 2009;3:1460–71. https://doi.org/10.1177/193229680900300628.

95. Dean AJ, Walters J, Hall A. A systematic review of interventions to enhance medication adherence in children and adolescents with chronic illness. Arch Dis Child. 2010;95:717–23. https://doi.org/10.1136/adc.2009.175125.

96. Graves MM, Roberts MC, Rapoff M, Boyer A. The efficacy of adherence interventions for chronically ill children: a meta-analytic review. J Pediatr Psychol. 2010;35:368–82. https://doi.org/10.1093/jpepsy/jsp072.

97. Barlow J, Wright C, Sheasby J, Turner A, Hainsworth J. Self-management approaches for people with chronic conditions: a review. Patient Educ Couns. 2002;48:177–87. https://doi.org/10.1016/s0738-3991(02)00032-0.

98. Lindsay S, Kolne K, Cagliostro E. Electronic mentoring programs and interventions for children and youth with disabilities: systematic review. JMIR Pediatr Parent. 2018;1(2):1–12. https://doi.org/10.2196/11679.

Self-Management Support for Young People with Chronic Conditions: Roles and Views of Professionals

Janet E. McDonagh

5.1   Introduction

All young people, as they grow up, ideally learn to self-manage their health within their capacity to do so. Supporting young people and their families in this process is integral to developmentally appropriate health care for all young people irrespective of health status. One of the key indicators of youth friendly health care identified in a systematic review of the literature addressing the young person's perspective, was young people being involved in their own health care which in turn was directly associated with a good understanding of their medical condition and treatment [1]. As an individual young person starts to take responsibility for their own healthcare, this is appropriately shared and supported by their parents/caregivers, family and friends. Autonomy development also needs to be supported by the health professionals they come into contact with and the services where they receive their health care. Self-management support is the support provided by healthcare professionals to young people and their family and other caregivers, so that young people can deal with the physical, emotional and social consequences of their chronic condition in daily life. In doing so, they develop self-confidence to sustain this health promoting behaviour for the rest of their life (adapted from [2]).

Addressing the transition to adulthood (including transfer) to adult healthcare is a key component of developmentally appropriate healthcare for all young people irrespective of health status. In two international and interdisciplinary Delphi studies involving health professionals, self-management was identified as an important

J. E. McDonagh (✉)
Versus Arthritis Centre for Epidemiology, Centre for Musculoskeletal Research, Faculty of Medical and Human Sciences, The University of Manchester, Manchester, UK

NIHR Manchester Musculoskeletal Biomedical Research Unit, Manchester University Hospitals NHS Foundations Trust, Manchester, UK

Manchester Academic Health Science Centre, Manchester, UK
e-mail: janet.mcdonagh@manchester.ac.uk

© Springer Nature Switzerland AG 2021
J. N. T. Sattoe et al. (eds.), *Self-Management of Young People with Chronic Conditions*, https://doi.org/10.1007/978-3-030-64293-8_5

outcome of transitional care for young people with chronic conditions [3, 4]. In one of these studies however, one could also argue that a further six outcomes identified are integral to medical self-management, namely disease knowledge, medical knowledge, adherence to treatment, understanding health insurance, attending medical appointments and avoidance of unnecessary hospitalisations [3]. In a prospective study of 374 young people with diabetes, cerebral palsy or autism spectrum disorder, promotion of young person's confidence in managing their health condition was one of three proposed beneficial features of transitional care services associated with better outcomes alongside appropriate parental involvement and meeting the adult health provider in advance [5]. However, only a fifth of participating centres in the study promoted such health self-efficacy. In another study of 8–16 year olds with asthma, health providers only obtained the young person's input into their asthma management treatment plan during 6% of encounters and caregiver input during only 10% of visits [6].

Adolescence and young adulthood has been recognised as a life stage with windows of opportunity to influence adult health as well as the health of the parents of tomorrow [7]. It is a life stage when both health promoting and health risk behaviours develop and when responsibility of management of health (and ill-health), influenced by such behaviours, moves from the caregiver to the individual young person. Furthermore, whereas in childhood when health services are accessed primarily by the caregivers on a child's behalf, during adolescence and young adulthood, young people become the "new users" of such services and start learning how to access and navigate services independently.

The aim of this chapter is to consider how healthcare professionals, health systems and the wider community can use this developmental window of opportunity to support and nurture self-management during adolescence and young adulthood.

5.2   Perspectives for the Health Professionals

5.2.1   Healthcare Professionals: The Individual

Healthcare professionals involved in the care of young people with chronic conditions are in a privileged position to support young people on their developmental journeys into adulthood. In the aforementioned systematic review of indicators of a youth friendly health service from the adolescent's perspective, a youth friendly healthcare provider was defined as "someone with accurate knowledge who could provide holistic care, was respectful and supportive, honest, trustworthy, and friendly" ([1], p. 678). Shaw et al. reported that provider characteristics are important determinants of adolescent satisfaction with transitional care [8]. It is therefore important for healthcare professionals to reflect on their own behaviours and attitudes with respect to this age group. Adolescence is a life stage when it is particularly important that individual healthcare professionals set aside any personal biases and prejudices with respect to this age group. In their professional lives, healthcare professionals need to acknowledge and separate any assumptions that are based on their own adolescence and those of their own children and/or relatives in addition to any sociocultural and religious backgrounds, thereby ensuring they are professionals first and foremost [9]. However, it is also important that services acknowledge the emotional impact of caring for young people with chronic conditions has on individual health of professionals, particularly at the time of transfer to adult care, and provide staff with appropriate and effective supervision [10].

5.2.2 Comparison of Health Priorities Between Professionals and Young People

In a Delphi study involving young people with Inflammatory Bowel Disease (IBD) and paediatric and adult gastroenterology professionals involved in their care, self-management skills were considered more important than IBD-specific items and there were no significant differences in ranking between respondent types [11]. However, in another study, there were significant discrepancies between perceived health priorities between young people with IBD and physicians, with physicians overestimating the worries of the young people and not acknowledging the impact of fatigue on their lives [12]. The authors of the latter study concluded that it is important to routinely asking young people the question: "what matters to you?", in order to truly understand the concerns of young people [13]. Relationships with healthcare professionals were identified as a key barrier and facilitator of self-management amongst adolescents with asthma [12]. Better self-management was reported when a positive relationship with the health professional was promoted and when the professional was competent, understanding and helpful [14, 15], echoing again the reported indicators of youth friendly services as perceived by young people [1].

5.2.3 Adjustment of Care as Young Person Grows Up

As in the rest of paediatrics, healthcare professionals have to learn to adjust as the young person develops, including when there is regression which can often happen in chronic conditions. This is also important for healthcare professionals involved with young people seen in the adult care setting where developmental assessments may be less routine. Chronological age is a poor predictor of developmental status [16, 17]. Moynihan et al. [16] reported that the strongest relationship with transition readiness as measured by Am I ONTRAC was the stage psychosocial development or maturity (i.e. the capacity to function independently and to interact with others outside of the family) [16]. Professionals who practice developmentally appropriate care and support appropriate youth autonomy have been reported to be the best to deliver transitional care [18]. Routine psychosocial screening and developmental assessment should be core to all consultations with young people. Psychosocial screening tools such as HEEADSSS (*H*ome, *E*ducation/*E*mployment, *E*ating, *A*ctivities, *D*rugs, *S*exuality, *S*uicidal ideation and mental health and *S*afety) [19] and THRxEADS (*T*ransition, *H*ome, *Rx* for Medication and Treatment, *E*ducation and Eating, *A*ctivities and Affect, *D*rugs and *S*exuality) [20] are useful in this regard both to engage the young person as well as to identify both protective as well as risk factors. Such protective factors include what resources, competencies, talents and skills young people already have which in turn both inform and be harnessed in the development of self-management strategies. How such tools are used in practice however may not always be effective. In a study of young people with a mean age of 17 years and the majority having a chronic condition, discrepancies were reported between what the young people recalled of the discussions of the HEEADSSS topics compared to what the health professional reported having discussed, particularly for the more sensitive of topics such as sexual health or mental health [21]. The findings raise questions regarding how the HEEADSSS questions were asked. Were they asked in a more interrogative than interactive manner? Was the timing appropriate? Had the professional engaged the young person? Was the young person ready to listen?

5.2.4 Relationships Between Professional and Young Person and/or Caregivers

Irrespective of setting, it is important to acknowledge the nature of both the relationship healthcare professionals have with the young person as well as with the parent/caregiver during adolescence [22]. The majority of parents provide ongoing emotional and practical support for their children irrespective of age. Hart et al. reported that parents/caregivers of young people with arthritis were still prominent players in decision-making around drug therapy into the third decade [23]. When a young person has a chronic condition which worsens or when the young person is distressed, parents can act as invaluable "safety nets" [24]. However, professionals also need to be aware of young people who may not have parents who can provide such support and may need this from trusted others as well as healthcare professionals.

Parents are key potential facilitators of their child's evolving self-management but their perceptions of their child's readiness, and competencies can impact, both positively and negatively on their child's progress to become managers of their own health [25, 26]. The needs of parents of young people with chronic conditions during adolescence and transition to adult-centred services are well described in the literature [25] though how best to address these has yet to be decided [27]. Supporting parents of young adults can sometimes be more challenging in an adult setting where there is more of a patient-centred rather than family-centred approach. In a study of 15–22 year olds with chronic conditions, some of whom would be in adult care, Peeters et al. [26] reported that parents were less convinced than their children regarding their autonomy than the young people themselves and tended to interfere in their daily lives often to the annoyance of their children. Healthcare professionals therefore may need to advocate for the young person whilst not alienating the parents. A core component of transitional care is educating parents about normal adolescent development and the need to promote skill development for their child's gradual evolving sense of autonomy. The role of parents is further discussed in Chap. 6.

5.2.5   Navigating Triadic Consultations

During adolescence, consultations are often triadic—involving the young person, their caregiver and the healthcare professionals. In spite of young people clearly wanting to be involved as partners in such consultations, their actual participation during consultations was low and neither requested nor encouraged with parents often filling the gap [28]. The different agendas—i.e. those of the young person, parent/caregiver, health professional—in the clinic room with respect to self-management therefore need to be acknowledged and negotiated by healthcare professionals as there can be discrepancies [12, 29, 30]. For example, the failure to engage in good self-care can be perceived by healthcare professionals as a skill deficit whereas the young person may perceive it is an active choice particularly when they have limited choice in the context of their chronic condition. A greater understanding of the young person's perspective can therefore lead to better informed interventions e.g. in the aforementioned scenario, self-care interventions would be better targeted at motivation rather than skills.

In a study of young people with a liver transplant, rejection was predicted by discrepancies between the respective perceptions of the young person and their parent/caregiver regarding self-management in addition to greater perceived self-management by the young person [29]. In another study of young people with diabetes, their parents/caregivers and their physicians, although all groups agreed that all self-care behaviours are important, there were key areas of discrepancy in perceptions, particularly between families and physicians [30]. Professionals need to acknowledge that their perception is influenced by their whole clinical practice of many individual patients and families whereas the young person and their family usually only have their own experience. Acknowledging and understanding these differing perceptions is important in order to improve the self-management and life skills of that individual young person.

In a study exploring self-management from the perspectives of youth, parents/caregivers and healthcare providers, Nguyen et al. [24] reported that a key theme was the perception of healthcare providers as enablers of and collaborators in self-management development [24]. Examples of how professionals can be enablers and collaborators within these triadic consultations are detailed in Table 5.1.

5.2.6   Differences Between Perceived and Actual Self-Management Skills

What is perceived as good self-management does not always translate into objective measures of good self-management. Fredericks et al. [31] reported that older adolescents (16–20 years) with liver transplants who reported greater perceived self-management had a greater risk for medication non-adherence [31]. Young adults with liver transplants reported health care self-management more often than adolescents, yet less than 50% of them demonstrated their skills i.e. did not manage their health care independently, did not make their own appointments and/or did not

Table 5.1 Examples of how healthcare professionals can facilitate and enable self-management training in clinic consultations

With young person	To facilitate communication between parent/caregiver and child
	To listen to the perspective of the young person
	To convey belief in young person
	To raise awareness of the developing strengths of the young person
	To raise awareness of the role the young person can play in their own health and well-being
	To motivate and assist the young person in taking on responsibility for their own health
	To actively promote the young person's strengths
With parents/ caregivers	To facilitate communication between parent/caregiver and child
	To listen to all perspectives
	To acknowledge discrepancies between these perspectives
	To convey belief and demonstrate competency of young person in the presence of the parent/caregiver
	To model respect towards young people in the presence of the parent/caregiver
	To identify and address parental needs
	To be an extra-parental adult and not a surrogate parent!

understand insurance issues [32]. Caution is required therefore when interpreting self-report-based measures.

This is further compounded by the fact that many self-management practices largely take place away from the clinic. The World Health Organisation's International Classification of Functioning distinguishes two features of the activities and participation components: namely, capacity and performance [33]. Capacity is the individual's ability to complete a task or action in a standardised environment like a clinic whereas performance is how well the individual is able to perform the task in their own environment [33]. Both capacity and performance need to be considered during discussions regarding self-management training. When capacity is greater than performance, potential barriers to self-management in the environment and personal contexts (such as motivation, self-efficacy, family influences) need to be considered.

5.2.7 Barriers and Facilitators to Self-Management

Healthcare professionals need to be cognizant of the barriers and facilitators to self-management [13]. Table 5.2 is a useful checklist for professionals of areas to cover in the assessment of self-management at routine clinic visits to identify such facilitators and barriers [13].

A key component of self-management training is communication between the young person and the various healthcare professionals involved in their care [13]. Health professional's communication skills and training in such skills have been reported to be associated with improved adherence [53]. A recent review

Table 5.2 Considerations when assessing self-management knowledge and skills

Knowledge of condition and therapy [15, 34–37]

Lifestyle influences e.g. daily routines, leisure activities, triggers, reminder cues [15, 34–43]

Beliefs and attitudes to health, condition and treatment [15, 34, 36–39, 41, 43]

Relationships with others (peers, teachers, healthcare professionals) [14, 15, 34–37, 40–42, 44, 45]

Intrapersonal characteristics e.g. motivation, feeling in control, potential for embarrassment [14, 34, 35, 39, 44–48]

Communication skills with respect to chronic condition including disclosure to friends, other professionals, future employers [15, 34, 37, 38, 49]

Opportunity for the young person to be seen independently of their parent/caregiver for at least part of each clinic visit [9]. When the caregivers return, the young person summarises the discussion and plan

Goal setting for self-care activities at home using information gathered with transition readiness tools [50, 51, 52]

considered how healthcare professionals can enhance their communication with young people to improve health outcomes [54]. Three themes were identified, namely: the challenges of addressing sensitive aspects the individual's life; trust and emotional safety as a prerequisite for effective communication; and the importance of young people being enabled to have a sense of inclusion and autonomy.

Croom et al. reported that adolescent-centred communication as perceived by the young person was positively associated with greater perceptions of control and competence of both adolescent and their parents/caregivers which in turn was associated with improved adherence and disease control [55]. The use of open-ended questions and emphasising the autonomy of the young person were reported to have most often led to change talk in a study considering which communication behaviours used by healthcare professionals predicted motivational statements in young people with obesity [56].

Bearing these in mind, potential solutions that healthcare professionals can use to enhance interpersonal communication with young people and thereby improve self-management knowledge and skills as well as other health outcomes have been summarised by Kim and White [54]. These solutions included the use of routine pathways and consultation tools to structure discussions; building trust and rapport first with explanations of why certain questions are being asked and having signposting and pathways to use, if issues are identified; and use of open-ended questions and shared decision-making. Kim and White [54] also highlighted that healthcare professionals need skills to assess competency, to promote autonomy appropriately, and to involve both the young person and their parent/caregiver appropriately—all vital skills to deliver self-management skills training.

There are many generic skills, integral to self-management, for which training can be readily incorporated and easily supported in routine clinical care. Such skills will also be invaluable for their future vocational lives as well—a useful rationale for such training to offer the young person and their parent/caregiver. Examples of these are detailed in Table 5.3.

Table 5.3 Generic skills of young people which health professionals can promote in consultations

Communication
Negotiation
Goal setting
Problem solving
Decision-making
Organisational skills (for example, planning)
Information seeking
Healthcare utilisation
Disclosure

Table 5.4 Considerations for facilitators of self-management skills training for young people at the multidisciplinary team level

Tracking of self-management skill acquisition of individual young people
Mechanisms of transition planning as a team
Consideration of team climate particularly at times of change
Shared policies and guideline-driven care to ensure consistency of approach
Continuity of professionals for individual young people when possible

5.2.8 Healthcare Professionals: The Team

Successful engagement of young people in transitional care requires a team-based approach [57]. A challenge for such multidisciplinary teams is communicating progress updates of individual young people within the team and thus coordinating self-management skills training and transitional care. Team-level issues for multidisciplinary teams providing transitional care for young people to consider are listed in Table 5.4.

Documentation of the tracking of the trajectories of such skill acquisition is important so that individual team members can build on what has already been achieved. There are various tools available to assist professionals to do this (see Chap. 8). One example of these are the Ready Steady Go communication tools [50] which adopted the individual plans developed with young people with arthritis in an earlier UK national transition study [51]. Following completion of a UK national transition research in rheumatology [51], an occupational therapist in one of the participating centres recognised the need to optimise the documentation of individual young people's progress within the wider multidisciplinary team and developed a team document to support the coordination of transitional care by the various members of the team [52]. This document has subsequently also been adopted by the Ready Steady Go programme [50]. It is sobering to note that in spite of the publication of the rheumatology research—it took nearly 10 years for wider adoption in the UK [50] and even yet, only 36.4% of European rheumatology centres use such tools and less than 10% use a specific readiness tool [58]. Similar results are reported in North America with 59% of 16–23 year olds with a range of chronic conditions in one study reporting no discussion of transition and 49% not yet seeing healthcare professionals independently for at least part of the visit [59].

There is a useful concept called the "team climate" which has been defined as a "team's shared perceptions of organisational policies, practices and procedures" [60]. Team climate and changes in team climate have been reported to predict the quality of transitional care delivery of which self-management is an integral component [61]. Consistency of approach is inherent to the team climate and shared policies addressing all areas of clinical practice are an important component of team working so that young people and their families do not receive "mixed messages". Such guidelines were highlighted as another key indicator of youth friendly health care as perceived by young people themselves [1]. Effective team working with young people with chronic conditions during adolescence however can be challenging particularly with respect to continuity and consistency of approach. Ideally, continuity of care by at least a couple of professionals should be aspired to, in order to enable trust to be established with individual young people. On average, it takes three to five visits before young people trust a health professional [62]. When continuity of staff is challenging, informational continuity with shared records and careful documentation increases in importance [63].

5.2.9 Healthcare Professionals in the Adult Care Setting

Due to the organisation of most health systems in developed countries, young people (10–24 year olds) are seen in both paediatric and adult care settings. As aforementioned, trajectories of transition skill acquisition such as self-management are recognised to exist over this lengthy developmental life stage [64, 65], with these trajectories being modified in the context of developmental disabilities and/or cognitive impairment. Stollon et al. [64] highlighted that although 50% of transition skills were acquired in early adolescence, the remaining 50% skills were acquired after 18 years of age and these skills included those relating to self-management, vocation, insurance, finding new healthcare professionals and reproductive health [64]. Similarly in a study of young people with Crohn's disease, by age 16–18 only 15% asked questions of the provider (males less likely) and by age 19–21 only 45% ordered medication refills (males less likely), 50% picked up medication from pharmacy, 35% scheduled appointments and only 30% contacted providers between visits if problems arose [65].

When gastroenterologists in adult healthcare were asked what the key aspects of transitional care from their perspective were, patient understanding of the disease itself and its therapy were high on the list [66, 67], as well as skills such as initiating contact if a problem arises in between appointments [66]. An interesting comparative study was conducted of adults with inflammatory bowel disease aged 25–55 years. In the latter study, 44% adults involved a family member/friend/spouse in picking up medications, 37% could not recall drug doses, 35% could not recall drug frequency and 73% on a biologic did not cite infection as a side effect [68]. This can perhaps be considered as evidence to support the concept of adolescence and young adulthood being a potential window of opportunity to influence such behaviours.

After the lengthy preparation phase of transition, comes the handover of care or transfer to adult service, which in turn is followed by the often forgotten third phase of transition which exists in adult care. The age at transfer to adult care is largely determined by chronological age rather than transition readiness [59], but coincides often with the move from shared to self-management as well as other social transitions such as educational and vocational transitions. A systematic review reported moderate evidence for models of transition which transfer young people in late adolescence or early adulthood to improve transition outcomes and patient satisfaction [69]. In acknowledgement of this third phase of transition, The Ready Steady Go Programme advocates the use of the "Hello to Adult services" list [50]. Several authors have advocated enhanced follow-up following transfer to ensure engagement of the young person in the third phase of transition [70]. In a study of young people with cystic fibrosis, Duguéperoux et al. [71] advised avoiding a long gap between last paediatric and first adult clinic appointment and to have at least 2–3 appointments with adult team in first year post transfer (irrespective of health status) to establish a therapeutic relationship [71]. In a more recent review of 1623 18–27 year olds with a range of chronic conditions in a single institution, clinics with higher proportions of successfully transferred patients had lower median numbers of days between last paediatric and first adult visit and higher transitional care quality scores [72]. When considering aspects of self-management related to health service utilisation, consideration of the youth friendliness and developmental appropriateness of the service provision is important. It may be the service which is influencing the performance even when the young person has the capacity (see above).

5.3 Perspectives for the Organisation

Healthcare professionals and multidisciplinary healthcare teams work within organisations. Likewise, young people rarely experience care in a single clinic setting and will often access other areas and services within and between organisations. It is therefore important to consider how self-management skills development and promotion is addressed at the organisation or system level. Modi and colleagues acknowledge this in the socio-ecological Paediatric Self-management Model which includes components representing the young person, their family, community and the health system [73] (see Chap. 3).

5.3.1 Developmentally Appropriate Healthcare

Adjustment of care as the young person develops in addition to the empowerment of the young person by embedding health education and health promotion have been identified as two of the five themes encompassed by the term developmentally appropriate healthcare (DAH) for young people [74]. However, in a qualitative multisite ethnographic study involving three hospitals in England and 192 professionals, there was a wide range of working definitions of DAH [52]. If the professionals involved in the care of young people cannot agree on what developmentally appropriate means, the question arises as to whether true DAH is actually being delivered in practice [75]. Interdisciplinary and intra-agency working was identified as one of the other dimensions of DAH, highlighting again the importance of considering such care beyond the one-to-one consultation. A toolkit resulting from this research is now available with specific guidance at clinic, team as well as at organisational levels [76].

5.3.2 Young Person Accessible and Responsive Services

One aspect of self-management is keeping appointments with healthcare professionals. Finding out the reason why young people do not attend is important as the reason is not always what professionals perceive as the reason. In a study of young people with cancer the common reason given was work and school conflicts [77]. Accessibility is a key system-based indicator of developmentally appropriate youth friendly care [1], e.g. having clinics only in the morning can be very limiting for young people in education with afternoon, twilight or evening clinics being preferable. In a study of young people with diabetes who did not attend clinics, it was a fear of being judged for "poor control" i.e. the high HbA1c that lead to their non-attendance and not vice versa [78]. Following on from this, how to chase up these "non-attenders" depends on whose contact details are kept on the hospital system. In paediatric hospitals it is often the parental details which are kept and therefore when a young person lives away from home, contacting them directly and learning why they did not attend can prove challenging. Likewise, if appointment letters are only sent to the parent/caregiver of the individual young person and not to the young person themselves, the young person may not feel acknowledged and therefore less motivated to remain engaged. Youth friendly services need to consider such practical aspects of the health administrative system during adolescence when responsibility for health and disease management begins to shift away from the parent/caregiver and towards the young person.

5.3.3 Adequate Time

One potential barrier to the delivery of self-management skills training in routine clinical care is lack of time particularly as the medical complexity of conditions and their therapies increase. Health systems need to acknowledge that clinic appointments with young people will take longer particularly if the young person comes with the parent [79]. In such cases, time needs to be allocated so that the young person can have some private time with the health professional as well as being seen with their parent/caregiver and any parental needs addressed. Frequency of appointments are also an important organisational consideration in the post transfer phase of transition once the young person is in the adult care settings as discussed above [48–50]. Nguyen et al. [24] highlighted the need for system level intervention such as adequate funding, institutional support and accreditation incentives to allow for designated time for healthcare providers to foster self-management skills in young people with chronic conditions and their parents/caregivers.

5.3.4 Learning to Navigate the Health System

As mentioned above, young people exist within the health system and not just within a single service and transitional and self-management knowledge and skills include those related to the ability to navigate such systems successfully. However, such health system knowledge is an underrepresented topic on some transition tools [58]. Involvement of the primary care physician is a core component of all transitional care guidance to date [79–81] although most of the research to date has focussed on specialty care providers. However, Han and colleagues reported that 34% of adolescents with chronic conditions had not seen their family physician in the previous 6 months and reported that some had a poor understanding of the family physician's role in coordinating care [82]. Knowing the "who" (e.g. family physician, emergency department), the why and the when of seeking help and advice is an important self-management skill and healthcare professionals should ensure such knowledge is included in self-management training programmes. It is important to remember the potential of all healthcare professionals in such information. For example, the potential role of the retail pharmacist is often underestimated and yet an invaluable and often more accessible member of the "team" for young people with chronic conditions [83].

Understanding how young people prefer to use health services is important as this is not always the same as adult counterparts. Often, we assume in this modern world that technology will always be the answer of adolescent focussed interventions and/or service provision. However, in a study of 13–21 year olds with chronic conditions, Applebaum and colleagues reported that, although young people preferred text messages to make appointments, they also admitted that they rarely checked voice mail nor email inboxes [84]. With respect to patient held records they disclosed that they were unlikely to take time for data entry unless fun and customisable. They were less interested in using social media to access information and communication with providers due to privacy concerns. The majority did not use computers or smart phones to store health-related info and rather relied on their parents/caregivers for this task [84]. It is therefore incumbent upon us as healthcare professionals to inquire and explore rather than assume knowledge of the world an individual young person lives in, if we are to support them effectively in becoming good self-managers of both their health as well as their chronic condition.

5.3.5 Workforce Competency

Finally, another key aspect of self-management at a system or organisation level is ensuring the workforce who supports self-management is competent to do so. The health care provider is a potential target for intervention to improve

Table 5.5 Considerations for facilitators of self-management skills training for young people at the health system levels

Developmentally appropriate healthcare
Young person accessible and responsive services
Adequate time e.g. clinic appointment duration, enhanced follow-up following transfer to adult care
Workforce competency

self-management amongst young people with chronic conditions. It is concerning that unmet training needs in adolescent health continue to be reported in both paediatric [85] and adult settings [86]. Attention to effective communication skills, psychosocial screening, developmental assessment, motivational interviewing skills and what constitutes developmentally appropriate healthcare for young people and youth friendly health services are core to such training. Considerations of self-management support at the team and health system levels are summarised in Table 5.5.

5.4   Perspectives for the Wider Community

To date, much of the research around self-management and transitional care has been focused on healthcare settings. However, young people live in a world beyond their immediate family and health care setting. A systematic review of the barriers and facilitators to self-management of asthma reported by adolescents concluded that "consideration of the wider social influences that impinge on self-management" was needed ([13], p. 430). The recent neuroscience advances with respect to social brain development, indicate that decision-making in adolescence may be particularly modulated by peers is of particular interest [87]; the role of peers is further discussed in Chap. 7.

Young people also need to self-manage their conditions in the world of education, training and/or work, whether it be disclosing their condition to employers or managing medication. Insensitive and/or unsupportive teachers as well as some school policies were identified as potential barriers to self-management in schools by young people with asthma [13]. Disclosure in the workplace is a major issue for young people with chronic conditions [88] and skills training not only in terms of both when and how to disclose but also the why and their rights under disability and equality legislation are important components of any self-management training.

In one of the few studies addressing the socio-ecological aspects of transition and self-management, Javalkar et al. [89] reported that the predictors of transition readiness/self-management included: local prevalence of females, median household income, and local prevalence of native speakers [89]. Attention to a social ecological model of self-management is therefore important [73] and routinely asking about home, peers, education/training/work and community environments in the assessment of shared and self-management practices during adolescence is important. Tools such as HEEADSSS [19] and THRxEADS [20] are useful to enable healthcare professionals to do this as part of routine psychosocial screening.

5.5   Key Recommendations for Practice

It has been known for many years that young people and their families need support as individual young people move from shared to self-management during adolescence and young adulthood [89]. However, suboptimal clinical practices continue to be reported [58, 59, 90] highlighting the need for further work as to understanding the barriers and facilitators in enabling young people to self-manage their health, their chronic condition as well as learn to navigate the health systems providing their care. Key recommendations are listed below:

1. Core components of training curricula of all healthcare professionals involved in the care of young people with chronic conditions in both paediatric and adult care settings are detailed in Table 5.6.
2. Self-management knowledge and skills training should be actively promoted at every encounter with a young person whilst acknowledging knowledge and skill acquisition will develop over time as the young person grows up. Tracking of these trajectories with appropriate documentation is vital to ensure appropriate involvement of individual team members and that progress is monitored. Clinic appointments need to acknowledge the time requirements for such training in addition to the other aspects of the appointment e.g. history taking, physical examination, treatment review, counselling, management planning, etc.
3. Self-management knowledge and skills training requires a team-based approach. However, multidisciplinary teams looking after such young people should ensure consistency of approach with written policies for how self-management training

Table 5.6 Core topics relevant to self-management support for training curricula of all Healthcare professionals involved in the care of young people

Knowledge	Adolescent and young adult biopsychosocial and cognitive development including the recent neuroscience advances and their implications on adolescent and young adult behaviour and decision-making [87, 91]
	Developmentally appropriate healthcare for young people [76]
	Youth friendly health service provision [1]
	Local resources and services for signposting
	Disclosure
Skills	Routine psychosocial assessment
	Routine developmental assessment
	Young person-centred communication skills
	Addressing health and illness beliefs
	Shared decision-making skills
	Motivational interviewing skills [92, 93]
	Health coaching skills

is delivered and enabled within the service, and tracking of these trajectories develops.

4. Self-management knowledge and skills training should be culturally competent and acknowledge the influences of cultural, religious, and ethnic backgrounds.

5. If language is a potential barrier, access to professional interpreters is important, both for delivery of information as well as assessment of knowledge and skills.

6. Healthcare professionals need to be aware of the interdependence of social and educational transitions on self-management and the rest of health transitions. Such stages can both represent a risk factor as well as the ideal timing for targeted intervention.

7. Active support of self-management for young people with chronic conditions needs to be considered at multiple levels: namely the one-to-one interaction with individual young people, interaction with their parent/caregivers, at a multidisciplinary team level and at a health system level.

5.6 Conclusion

This chapter has highlighted the important role healthcare professionals, health systems and the wider community have in enabling, supporting and nurturing self-management practice development during adolescence and young adulthood. This particular life stage is a developmental window of opportunity to do this and healthcare professionals involved with such young people need to be trained in order to do this.

Acknowledgements Supported by Versus Arthritis Centre for Epidemiology (UK grant No: R122049) and the NIHR Manchester Biomedical Research Centre.

References

1. Ambresin AE, Bennett K, Patton GC, Sanci LA, Sawyer SM. Assessment of youth-friendly health care: a systematic review of indicators drawn from young people's perspectives. J Adolesc Health. 2013;52(6):670–81. https://doi.org/10.1016/j.jadohealth.2012.12.014.

2. Bodenheimer T, Lorig K, Holman H, Grumbach K. Patient self-management of chronic disease in primary care. JAMA. 2002;288(19):2469–75. https://doi.org/10.1001/jama.288.19.2469.

3. Fair C, Cuttance J, Sharma N, Maslow G, Wiener L, Betz C, Porter J, McLaughlin S, Gilleland-Marchak J, Renwick A, Naranjo D, Jan S, Javalkar K, Ferris M, International and Interdisciplinary Health Care Transition Research Consortium. International and interdisciplinary identification of health care transition outcomes. JAMA Pediatr. 2016;170(3):205–11. https://doi.org/10.1001/jamapediatrics.2015.3168.

4. Surís JC, Akré C. Key elements for, and indicators of, a successful transition: an international Delphi study. J Adolesc Health. 2015;56(6):612–8. https://doi.org/10.1016/j.jadohealth.2015.02.007.

5. Colver A, McConachie H, Le Couteur A, Dovey-Pearce G, Mann KD, McDonagh JE, Pearce MS, Vale L, Merrick H, Parr JR, Transition Collaborative Group. A longitudinal, observational study of the features of transitional healthcare associated with better outcomes for

young people with long-term conditions. BMC Med. 2018;16(1):111. https://doi.org/10.1186/s12916-018-1102-y.

6. Sleath BL, Carpenter DM, Sayner R, Ayala GX, Williams D, Davis S, Tudor G, Yeatts K. Child and caregiver involvement and shared decision-making during asthma pediatric visits. J Asthma. 2011;48(10):1022–31. https://doi.org/10.3109/02770903.2011.626482.

7. Patton GC, Olsson CA, Skirbekk V, Saffery R, Wlodek ME, Azzopardi PS, Stonawski M, Rasmussen B, Spry E, Francis K, Bhutta ZA, Kassebaum NJ, Mokdad AH, Murray C, Prentice AM, Reavley N, Sheehan P, Sweeny K, Viner RM, Sawyer SM. Adolescence and the next generation. Nature. 2018;554(7693):458–66. https://doi.org/10.1038/nature25759.

8. Shaw KL, Southwood TR, McDonagh JE, British Society of Paediatric and Adolescent Rheumatology. Young people's satisfaction of transitional care in adolescent rheumatology in the UK. Child Care Health Dev. 2007;33(4):368–79. https://doi.org/10.1111/j.1365-2214.2006.00698.x.

9. McDonagh JE, Kaufman M. The challenging adolescent. Rheumatology (Oxford). 2009;48(8):872–5. https://doi.org/10.1093/rheumatology/kep133.

10. Wright J, Elwell L, McDonagh J, Kelly D, McClean P, Ferguson J, Wray J. Healthcare transition in pediatric liver transplantation: the perspectives of pediatric and adult healthcare professionals. Pediatr Transplant. 2019;23(6):e13530. https://doi.org/10.1111/petr.13530.

11. van den Brink G, van Gaalen M, de Ridder L, van der Woude CJ, Escher JC. Health care transition outcomes in inflammatory bowel disease: a multinational delphi study. J Crohns Colitis. 2019;13(9):1163–72. https://doi.org/10.1093/ecco-jcc/jjz044.

12. Cervesi C, Battistutta S, Martelossi S, Ronfani L, Ventura A. Health priorities in adolescents with inflammatory bowel disease: physicians' versus patients' perspectives. J Pediatr Gastroenterol Nutr. 2013;57(1):39–42. https://doi.org/10.1097/MPG.0b013e31828b5fd4.

13. Holley S, Morris R, Knibb R, Latter S, Liossi C, Mitchell F, Roberts G. Barriers and facilitators to asthma self-management in adolescents: a systematic review of qualitative and quantitative studies. Pediatr Pulmonol. 2017;52(4):430–42. https://doi.org/10.1002/ppul.23556.

14. Jonsson M, Egmar AC, Hallner E, Kull I. Experiences of living with asthma - a focus group study with adolescents and parents of children with asthma. J Asthma. 2014;51(2):185–92. https://doi.org/10.3109/02770903.2013.853080.

15. Wamboldt FS, Bender BG, Rankin AE. Adolescent decision-making about use of inhaled asthma controller medication: results from focus groups with participants from a prior longitudinal study. J Asthma. 2011;48(7):741–50. https://doi.org/10.3109/02770903.2011.598204.

16. Moynihan M, Saewyc E, Whitehouse S, Paone M, McPherson G. Assessing readiness for transition from paediatric to adult health care: revision and psychometric evaluation of the Am I ON TRAC for Adult Care questionnaire. J Adv Nurs. 2015;71(6):1324–35. https://doi.org/10.1111/jan.12617.

17. Paine CW, Stollon NB, Lucas MS, Brumley LD, Poole ES, Peyton T, Grant AW, Jan S, Trachtenberg S, Zander M, Mamula P, Bonafide CP, Schwartz LA. Barriers and facilitators to successful transition from pediatric to adult inflammatory bowel disease care from the perspectives of providers. Inflamm Bowel Dis. 2014;20(11):2083–91. https://doi.org/10.1097/MIB.0000000000000136.

18. Wells CK, McMorris BJ, Horvath KJ, Garwick AW, Scal PB. Youth report of healthcare transition counseling and autonomy support from their rheumatologist. Pediatr Rheumatol Online J. 2012;10(1):36. https://doi.org/10.1186/1546-0096-10-36.

19. Doukrou M, Segal TY. Fifteen-minute consultation: communicating with young people-how to use HEEADSSS, a psychosocial interview for adolescents. Archiv Dis Childhood Educ Pract. 2018;103(1):15–9. https://doi.org/10.1136/archdischild-2016-311553.

20. Chadi N, Amaria K, Kaufman M. Expand your HEADS, follow the THRxEADS! Paediatr Child Health. 2017;22(1):23–5. https://doi.org/10.1093/pch/pxw007.

21. Boisen KA, Hertz PG, Blix C, Teilmann G. Is HEADS in our heads? Health risk behavior is not routinely discussed with young people with chronic conditions. Int J Adolesc Med Health. 2016;28(4):429–35. https://doi.org/10.1515/ijamh-2015-0015.

22. Ford CA, Davenport AF, Meier A, McRee AL. Partnerships between parents and health care professionals to improve adolescent health. J Adolesc Health. 2011;49(1):53–7. https://doi.org/10.1016/j.jadohealth.2010.10.004.
23. Hart RI, Foster HE, McDonagh JE, Thompson B, Kay L, Myers A, Rapley T. Young people's decisions about biologic therapies: who influences them and how? Rheumatology (Oxford). 2015;54(7):1294–301. https://doi.org/10.1093/rheumatology/keu523.
24. Nguyen T, Henderson D, Stewart D, Hlyva O, Punthakee Z, Gorter JW. You never transition alone! Exploring the experiences of youth with chronic health conditions, parents and healthcare providers on self-management. Child Care Health Dev. 2016;42(4):464–72. https://doi.org/10.1111/cch.12334.
25. Heath G, Farre A, Shaw K. Parenting a child with chronic illness as they transition into adulthood: a systematic review and thematic synthesis of parents' experiences. Patient Educ Couns. 2017;100(1):76–92. https://doi.org/10.1016/j.pec.2016.08.011.
26. Peeters MA, Hilberink SR, van Staa A. The road to independence: lived experiences of youth with chronic conditions and their parents compared. J Pediatr Rehabil Med. 2014;7(1):33–42. https://doi.org/10.3233/PRM-140272.
27. Akré C, Ramelet AS, Berchtold A, Surís JC. Educational intervention for parents of adolescents with chronic illness: a pre-post test pilot study. Int J Adolesc Med Health. 2015;27(3):261–9. https://doi.org/10.1515/ijamh-2014-0020.
28. van Staa A, On Your Own Feet Research Group. Unraveling triadic communication in hospital consultations with adolescents with chronic conditions: the added value of mixed methods research. Patient Educ Couns. 2011;82(3):455–64. https://doi.org/10.1016/j.pec.2010.12.001.
29. Annunziato RA, Bucuvalas JC, Yin W, Arnand R, Alonso EM, Mazariegos GV, Venick RS, Stuber ML, Shneider BL, Shemesh E. Self-management measurement and prediction of clinical outcomes in pediatric transplant. J Pediatr. 2018;193:128–133.e2. https://doi.org/10.1016/j.jpeds.2017.09.069.
30. Palladino DK, Helgeson VS. Adolescents, parents and physicians: a comparison of perspectives on type 1 diabetes self-care. Can J Diabetes. 2013;37(3):175–81. https://doi.org/10.1016/j.jcjd.2013.02.057.
31. Fredericks EM, Dore-Stites D, Well A, Magee JC, Freed GL, Shieck V, James Lopez M. Assessment of transition readiness skills and adherence in pediatric liver transplant recipients. Pediatr Transplant. 2010;14(8):944–53. https://doi.org/10.1111/j.1399-3046.2010.01349.x.
32. Annunziato RA, Parkar S, Dugan CA, Barsade S, Arnon R, Miloh T, Iyer K, Kerkar N, Shemesh E. Brief report: deficits in health care management skills among adolescent and young adult liver transplant recipients transitioning to adult care settings. J Pediatr Psychol. 2011;36(2):155–9. https://doi.org/10.1093/jpepsy/jsp110.
33. Almansa J, Ayuso-Mateos JL, Garin O, Chatterji S, Kostanjsek N, Alonso J, Valderas JM, Cieza A, Raggi A, Svestkova O, Burger H, Racca V, Vieta E, Leonardi M, Ferrer M, MHADIE Consortium. The international classification of functioning, disability and health: development of capacity and performance scales. J Clin Epidemiol. 2011;64(12):1400–11. https://doi.org/10.1016/j.jclinepi.2011.03.005.
34. Edgecombe K, Latter S, Peters S, Roberts G. Health experiences of adolescents with uncontrolled severe asthma. Arch Dis Child. 2010;95(12):985–91. https://doi.org/10.1136/adc.2009.171579.
35. Rhee H, Belyea MJ, Ciurzynski S, Brasch J. Barriers to asthma self-management in adolescents: relationships to psychosocial factors. Pediatr Pulmonol. 2009;44(2):183–91. https://doi.org/10.1002/ppul.20972.
36. Buston KM, Wood SF. Non-compliance amongst adolescents with asthma: listening to what they tell us about self-management. Fam Pract. 2000;17(2):134–8. https://doi.org/10.1093/fampra/17.2.134.
37. Velsor-Friedrich B, Vlasses F, Moberley J, Coover L. Talking with teens about asthma management. J Sch Nurs. 2004;20(3):140–8. https://doi.org/10.1177/10598405040200030401.

38. van Es SM, le Coq EM, Brouwer AI, Mesters I, Nagelkerke AF, Colland VT. Adherence-related behavior in adolescents with asthma: results from focus group interviews. J Asthma. 1998;35(8):637–46. https://doi.org/10.3109/02770909809048966.
39. Naimi DR, Freedman TG, Ginsburg KR, Bogen D, Rand CS, Apter AJ. Adolescents and asthma: why bother with our meds? J Allergy Clin Immunol. 2009;123(6):1335–41. https://doi.org/10.1016/j.jaci.2009.02.022.
40. Blaakman SW, Cohen A, Fagnano M, Halterman JS. Asthma medication adherence among urban teens: a qualitative analysis of barriers, facilitators and experiences with school-based care. J Asthma. 2014;51(5):522–9. https://doi.org/10.3109/02770903.2014.885041.
41. Koster ES, Philbert D, de Vries TW, van Dijk L, Bouvy ML. "I just forget to take it": asthma self-management needs and preferences in adolescents. J Asthma. 2015;52(8):831–7. https://doi.org/10.3109/02770903.2015.1020388.
42. Knight D. Beliefs and self-care practices of adolescents with asthma. Issues Compr Pediatr Nurs. 2005;28(2):71–81. https://doi.org/10.1080/01460860590950845.
43. van Es SM, Kaptein AA, Bezemer PD, Nagelkerke AF, Colland VT, Bouter LM. Predicting adherence to prophylactic medication in adolescents with asthma: an application of the ASE-model. Patient Educ Couns. 2002;47(2):165–71. https://doi.org/10.1016/s0738-3991(01)00195-1.
44. Araújo A, Rocha RL, Alvim CG. Adolescência e manejo da asma: a perspectiva dos assistidos na atenção primária à saúde [Adolescence and asthma management: the perspective of adolescents receiving primary health care]. Revista Paulista de Pediatria. 2014;32(3):171–6. https://doi.org/10.1590/0103-0582201432304.
45. Kyngas HA. Nurses' support: essential factor for the good compliance of adolescents with asthma. Nurs Health Sci. 2000;2(4):211–6. https://doi.org/10.1046/j.1442-2018.2000.00060.x.
46. van Es SM, Nagelkerke AF, Colland VT, Scholten RJ, Bouter LM. An intervention programme using the ASE-model aimed at enhancing adherence in adolescents with asthma. Patient Educ Couns. 2001;44(3):193–203. https://doi.org/10.1016/s0738-3991(00)00195-6.
47. Cohen R, Franco K, Motlow F, Reznik M, Ozuah PO. Perceptions and attitudes of adolescents with asthma. J Asthma. 2003;40(2):207–11. https://doi.org/10.1081/jas-120017992.
48. Quaranta J, Wool M, Logvis K, Brown K, Joshy D. Interpersonal influences on the self-management skills of the rural asthmatic adolescent. Online J Rural Nurs Health Care. 2014;14:97–122. https://doi.org/10.14574/ojrnhc.v14i2.281.
49. Mammen J, Rhee H. Adolescent asthma self-management: a concept analysis and operational definition. Pediatr Allergy Immunol Pulmonol. 2012;25(4):180–9. https://doi.org/10.1089/ped.2012.0150.
50. Nagra A, McGinnity PM, Davis N, Salmon AP. Implementing transition: ready steady go. Archiv Dis Childhood Educ Pract. 2015;100(6):313–20. https://doi.org/10.1136/archdischild-2014-307423.
51. McDonagh JE, Shaw KL, Southwood TR. Growing up and moving on in rheumatology: development and preliminary evaluation of a transitional care programme for a multicentre cohort of adolescents with juvenile idiopathic arthritis. J Child Health Care. 2006;10(1):22–42. https://doi.org/10.1177/1367493506060203.
52. McDonagh JE, Hackett J, McGee M, Southwood T, Shaw KL. The evidence base for transition is bigger than you might think. Archiv Dis Childhood Educ Pract. 2015;100(6):321–2. https://doi.org/10.1136/archdischild-2015-309204.
53. Zolnierek KB, Dimatteo MR. Physician communication and patient adherence to treatment: a meta-analysis. Med Care. 2009;47(8):826–34. https://doi.org/10.1097/MLR.0b013e31819a5acc.
54. Kim B, White K. How can health professionals enhance interpersonal communication with adolescents and young adults to improve health care outcomes? Systematic literature review. Int J Adolesc Youth. 2017;23(2):198–218. https://doi.org/10.1080/02673843.2017.1330696.
55. Croom A, Wiebe DJ, Berg CA, Lindsay R, Donaldson D, Foster C, Murray M, Swinyard MT. Adolescent and parent perceptions of patient-centered communication while managing type 1 diabetes. J Pediatr Psychol. 2011;36(2):206–15. https://doi.org/10.1093/jpepsy/jsq072.

56. Carcone AI, Naar-King S, Brogan KE, Albrecht T, Barton E, Foster T, Martin T, Marshall S. Provider communication behaviors that predict motivation to change in black adolescents with obesity. J Dev Behav Pediatr. 2013;34(8):599–608. https://doi.org/10.1097/DBP.0b013e3182a67daf.
57. van Staa A, Sattoe JN, Strating MM. Experiences with and outcomes of two interventions to maximize engagement of chronically ill adolescents during hospital consultations: a mixed methods study. J Pediatr Nurs. 2015;30(5):757–75. https://doi.org/10.1016/j.pedn.2015.05.028.
58. Clemente D, Leon L, Foster H, Carmona L, Minden K. Transitional care for rheumatic conditions in Europe: current clinical practice and available resources. Pediatr Rheumatol Online J. 2017;15(1):49. https://doi.org/10.1186/s12969-017-0179-8.
59. Jensen PT, Paul GV, LaCount S, Peng J, Spencer CH, Higgins GC, Boyle B, Kamboj M, Smallwood C, Ardoin SP. Assessment of transition readiness in adolescents and young adults with chronic health conditions. Pediatr Rheumatol Online J. 2017;15(1):70. https://doi.org/10.1186/s12969-017-0197-6.
60. Anderson N, West MA. Measuring climate for work group innovation: development and validation of the team climate inventory. J Organ Behav. 1998;19:235–58.
61. Cramm JM, Strating MM, Nieboer AP. The role of team climate in improving the quality of chronic care delivery: a longitudinal study among professionals working with chronically ill adolescents in transitional care programmes. BMJ Open. 2014;4(5):e005369. https://doi.org/10.1136/bmjopen-2014-005369.
62. Klostermann BK, Slap GB, Nebrig DM, Tivorsak TL, Britto MT. Earning trust and losing it: adolescents' views on trusting physicians. J Fam Pract. 2005;54(8):679–87.
63. Allen D, Cohen D, Hood K, Robling M, Atwell C, Lane C, Lowes L, Channon S, Gillespie D, Groves S, Harvey J, Gregory J. Continuity of care in the transition from child to adult diabetes services: a realistic evaluation study. J Health Serv Res Policy. 2012;17(3):140–8. https://doi.org/10.1258/JHSRP.2011.011044.
64. Stollon N, Zhong Y, Ferris M, Bhansali S, Pitts B, Rak E, Kelly M, Kim S, van Tilburg M. Chronological age when healthcare transition skills are mastered in adolescents/young adults with inflammatory bowel disease. World J Gastroenterol. 2017;23(18):3349–55. https://doi.org/10.3748/wjg.v23.i18.3349.
65. van Groningen J, Ziniel S, Arnold J, Fishman LN. When independent healthcare behaviors develop in adolescents with inflammatory bowel disease. Inflamm Bowel Dis. 2012;18(12):2310–4. https://doi.org/10.1002/ibd.22937.
66. Barendse RM, van de Kerk DJ, Fishman LN, Grand RJ, Bartelsman JF, Heymans HAS. Transition of adolescents with inflammatory bowel disease from pediatric to adult care: a survey of Dutch adult gastroenterologists' perspectives. Int J Child Adolesc Health. 2011;3(4):609–16. https://doi.org/10.1097/MPG.0b013e31816d71d8.
67. Hait EJ, Barendse RM, Arnold JH, Valim C, Sands BE, Korzenik JR, Fishman LN. Transition of adolescents with inflammatory bowel disease from pediatric to adult care: a survey of adult gastroenterologists. J Pediatr Gastroenterol Nutr. 2009;48(1):61–5. https://doi.org/10.1097/MPG.0b013e31816d71d8.
68. Fishman LN, Mitchell PD, Lakin PR, Masciarelli L, Flier SN. Are expectations too high for transitioning adolescents with inflammatory bowel disease? Examining adult medication knowledge and self-management skills. J Pediatr Gastroenterol Nutr. 2016;63(5):494–9. https://doi.org/10.1097/MPG.0000000000001299.
69. Yassaee A, Hale D, Armitage A, Viner R. The impact of age of transfer on outcomes in the transition from pediatric to adult health systems: a systematic review of reviews. J Adolesc Health. 2019;64(6):709–20. https://doi.org/10.1016/j.jadohealth.2018.11.023.
70. Crowley R, Wolfe I, Lock K, McKee M. Improving the transition between paediatric and adult healthcare: a systematic review. Arch Dis Child. 2011;96(6):548–53. https://doi.org/10.1136/adc.2010.202473.
71. Duguéperoux I, Tamalet A, Sermet-Gaudelus I, Le Bourgeois M, Gérardin M, Desmazes-Dufeu N, Hubert D. Clinical changes of patients with cystic fibrosis during transition from

pediatric to adult care. J Adolesc Health. 2008;43(5):459–65. https://doi.org/10.1016/j.jadohealth.2008.03.005.

72. Hart LC, Patel-Nguyen SV, Merkley MG, Jonas DE. An evidence map for interventions addressing transition from pediatric to adult care: a systematic review of systematic reviews. J Pediatr Nurs. 2019;48:18–34. https://doi.org/10.1016/j.pedn.2019.05.015.

73. Modi AC, Pai AL, Hommel KA, Hood KK, Cortina S, Hilliard ME, Guilfoyle SM, Gray WN, Drotar D. Pediatric self-management: a framework for research, practice, and policy. Pediatrics. 2012;129(2):e473–85. https://doi.org/10.1542/peds.2011-1635.

74. Farre A, Wood V, McDonagh JE, Parr JR, Reape D, Rapley T, Transition Collaborative Group. Health professionals' and managers' definitions of developmentally appropriate healthcare for young people: conceptual dimensions and embedded controversies. Arch Dis Child. 2016;101(7):628–33. https://doi.org/10.1136/archdischild-2015-309473.

75. Rapley T, Farre A, Parr JR, Wood VJ, Reape D, Dovey-Pearce G, McDonagh J, Transition Collaborative Group. Can we normalise developmentally appropriate health care for young people in UK hospital settings? An ethnographic study. BMJ Open. 2019;9(9):e029107. https://doi.org/10.1136/bmjopen-2019-029107.

76. McDonagh JE, Farre A, Gleeson H, Rapley T, Dovey-Pearce G, Reape D, Rigby E, Colver AF, Parr JR, Transition Collaborative Group. Making healthcare work for young people. Arch Dis Child. 2018;103(6):623. https://doi.org/10.1136/archdischild-2017-314573.

77. Klosky JL, Cash DK, Buscemi J, Lensing S, Garces-Webb DM, Zhao W, Wiard S, Hudson MM. Factors influencing long-term follow-up clinic attendance among survivors of child-hood cancer. J Cancer Surviv Res Pract. 2008;2(4):225–32. https://doi.org/10.1007/s11764-008-0063-0.

78. Snow R, Fulop N. Understanding issues associated with attending a young adult diabetes clinic: a case study. Diabet Med. 2012;29(2):257–9. https://doi.org/10.1111/j.1464-5491.2011.03447.x.

79. Royal College of Paediatrics and Child Health. Facing the future: standards for children with ongoing health needs. 2018. https://www.rcpch.ac.uk/resources/facing-future-standards-ongoing-health-needs. Accessed 3 April 2020.

80. Bhawra J, Toulany A, Cohen E, Moore Hepburn C, Guttmann A. Primary care interventions to improve transition of youth with chronic health conditions from paediatric to adult healthcare: a systematic review. BMJ Open. 2016;6(5):e011871. https://doi.org/10.1136/bmjopen-2016-011871.

81. Foster HE, Minden K, Clemente D, Leon L, McDonagh JE, Kamphuis S, Berggren K, van Pelt P, Wouters C, Waite-Jones J, Tattersall R, Wyllie R, Stones SR, Martini A, Constantin T, Schalm S, Fidanci B, Erer B, Demirkaya E, Ozen S, et al. EULAR/PReS standards and recommendations for the transitional care of young people with juvenile-onset rheumatic diseases. Ann Rheum Dis. 2017;76(4):639–46. https://doi.org/10.1136/annrheumdis-2016-210112.

82. Han AX, Whitehouse SR, Tsai S, Hwang S, Thorne S. Perceptions of the family physician from adolescents and their caregivers preparing to transition to adult care. BMC Fam Pract. 2018;19(1):140. https://doi.org/10.1186/s12875-018-0830-6.

83. Gray NJ, Shaw KL, Smith FJ, Burton J, Prescott J, Roberts R, Terry D, McDonagh JE. The role of pharmacists in caring for young people with chronic illness. J Adolesc Health. 2017;60(2):219–25. https://doi.org/10.1016/j.jadohealth.2016.09.023.

84. Applebaum MA, Lawson EF, von Scheven E. Perception of transition readiness and preferences for use of technology in transition programs: teens' ideas for the future. Int J Adolesc Med Health. 2013;25(2):119–25. https://doi.org/10.1515/ijamh-2013-0019.

85. Michaud PA, Jansen D, Schrier L, Vervoort J, Visser A, Dembiński Ł. An exploratory survey on the state of training in adolescent medicine and health in 36 European countries. Eur J Pediatr. 2019;178(10):1559–65. https://doi.org/10.1007/s00431-019-03445-1.

86. Wright RJ, Howard EJ, Newbery N, Gleeson H. 'Training gap' - the present state of higher specialty training in adolescent and young adult health in medical specialties in the UK. Fut Healthcare J. 2017;4(2):80–95. https://doi.org/10.7861/futurehosp.4-2-80.

87. Blakemore SJ, Robbins TW. Decision-making in the adolescent brain. Nat Neurosci. 2012;15(9):1184–91. https://doi.org/10.1038/nn.3177.

88. Farre A, Ryan S, McNiven A, McDonagh JE. The impact of arthritis on the educational and early work experiences of young people: a qualitative secondary analysis. Int J Adolesc Med Health. 2019; https://doi.org/10.1515/ijamh-2018-0240.
89. Javalkar K, Johnson M, Kshirsagar AV, Ocegueda S, Detwiler RK, Ferris M. Ecological factors predict transition readiness/self-management in youth with chronic conditions. J Adolesc Health. 2016;58(1):40–6. https://doi.org/10.1016/j.jadohealth.2015.09.013.
90. Kieckhefer GM, Trahms CM. Supporting development of children with chronic conditions: from compliance toward shared management. Pediatr Nurs. 2000;26(4):354–63.
91. Colver A, Longwell S. New understanding of adolescent brain development: relevance to transitional healthcare for young people with long term conditions. Arch Dis Child. 2013;98(11):902–7. https://doi.org/10.1136/archdischild-2013-303945.
92. Caccavale LJ, Corona R, LaRose JG, Mazzeo SE, Sova AR, Bean MK. Exploring the role of motivational interviewing in adolescent patient-provider communication about type 1 diabetes. Pediatr Diabetes. 2019;20(2):217–25. https://doi.org/10.1111/pedi.12810.
93. Naar-King S, Suarez M. Motivational interviewing with adolescents and young adults. New York, NY: Guildford Press; 2011.

Karen L. Shaw, Gemma Heath, and Albert Farre

6.1 Introduction

Transitional care is that which is provided by parents and health professionals throughout adolescence and emerging adulthood. It is characterised as a time of change whereby young people move towards assuming responsibility for their chronic condition, in line with their development and in preparation for the transition to adulthood and adult healthcare services.

For many years, parents were either absent from the transitional care literature or conceptualised as a barrier to young people's independence; a view that still pervades contemporary narratives. More recently, there has been a discernible shift that repositions parents as key enablers in transition and protective factors in young people's health and wellbeing. This positive stance is increasingly reflected in policies for transitional care, which now define parents as legitimate stakeholders, key informants and service users. These recognise that parents have an influential role in young people's health and development. However, they also acknowledge that parents are widely critical of care provision during transition. Improving parental support is, therefore, an explicit priority for service improvement. Unfortunately, while policy makers are keen to drive-up standards in care, they provide scant detail about what effective parenting in transition looks like, or how to support families in transferring caring responsibilities for optimal benefit.

In response, this chapter brings together the latest evidence about parenting in the context of transition. In doing so, we make an important distinction—that

K. L. Shaw (✉)
Institute of Applied Health Research, University of Birmingham, Birmingham, UK
e-mail: k.l.shaw@bham.ac.uk

G. Heath
Department of Psychology, University of Wolverhampton, Wolverhampton, UK

A. Farre
School of Health Sciences, University of Dundee, Dundee, UK

© Springer Nature Switzerland AG 2021
J. N. T. Sattoe et al. (eds.), *Self-Management of Young People with Chronic Conditions*, https://doi.org/10.1007/978-3-030-64293-8_6

107

parents are involved in two interrelated transitions: (1) the transfer of healthcare responsibility from parents to young people — *health transition* and (2) the relocation of young people's healthcare services from paediatric to adult providers — *transitional care* [1].

The first part, *Parenting in Transition*, explores what it means to be a parent of a young person with a chronic condition during health transition. This explains why transition cannot be understood as a young person-only phenomenon. We then draw upon existing literature to demonstrate how parents and young people can, and do, work together to shape the emotional environments necessary for positive realignment of roles and responsibilities. This highlights the potential of parents to play beneficial and protective roles in young people's transition, rather than problematizing parenting, which has historically been the case. However, we also reveal the unmet support needs of parents that place them and their children at risk of poor outcomes. Drawing upon psychological theory, we discuss why a 'whole family approach' is now warranted.

The second part, *Parenting and Transitional Care*, examines parental roles in relation to service provision and the adequacy of current arrangements to offer meaningful support. We discuss the different ways in which parenting has been conceptualised in relation to adolescent health (generally) and transitional care (specifically). In doing so, we explore a strengths-based approach that views parents as assets in transitional care; arguing that improving parental capabilities will benefit young people's health, wellbeing and transition readiness. We highlight a number of ways to foster positive relationships with parents in transitional care settings and challenge the prevailing view that young people are expected to manage their condition independently.

The final part, *Key Recommendations for Practice* presents a range of evidence-based strategies to accommodate family support appropriately throughout paediatric and adult healthcare, including priorities for research and development.

At this point, it is important to note that the term 'parent/s' is used in this chapter as an umbrella term to include all primary caregivers responsible for parenting during transition, which includes (but is not limited to) biological parents, other guardians such as step-parents and foster parents, and other adult family members such as grandparents and older siblings.

6.2　Parenting in Transition

It is expected that children will incrementally increase responsibility for managing their chronic condition as they move through adolescence and into adulthood. This usually involves a shift from parental to shared responsibility, followed by a shift to young people themselves, where capacity allows [2–4]. For parents, this represents a change in their role from 'care provider' to that of 'care consultant' [5], while embedding this new role within an adult-adult relationship [6]. This realignment of roles and responsibilities is central to the Shared Management Model (introduced in Chap. 3) which is enacted within clinical contexts, but evolves as part of everyday family life.

Studies examining the changing roles of parents during transition [1, 6–12] conceptualise the problem as: adaptation to a marginalised role, appropriate allocation of treatment responsibilities and managing anxieties related to their child's illness trajectory [13–15]. It is unsurprising, therefore, that effective change from parental management to self-management is tricky. It requires fine balancing [8, 10, 13, 15] and sharing care is both a source of support and conflict for young people and their parents [2, 4, 9, 13, 16–18]. Getting the balance right is important; having too little responsibility for self-care or being 'forced' to take on responsibility prematurely can impact on young people's health and use of healthcare, including non-compliance, missed appointments and delays in transfer [19]. Thus, there is much need to understand how parents and young people can be supported to manage the shift in responsibilities, starting with a better understanding of the roles that parents play in young people's transition readiness. This section therefore draws together research that describes the supporting roles that parents perform in their children's transition and the impact this can have on their own health, wellbeing and personal development. It also demonstrates how parents understand their changing roles and responsibilities, explaining why they enact them as they do. Importantly, this includes evidence from parents themselves (e.g. [4]).

6.2.1 Experiences and Impact of Parenting in Transition

Typically, parents hold a number of roles and responsibilities in transition; not least functioning as scaffolds, supporting young people to develop the skills they need to become independent and effective health service users. Where there are complex health conditions and additional care needs, these roles have been shown to be intensified and extended to include the roles of nurse, student, teacher, detective, guard, advocate [20]. Parenting roles in transition have also been shown to extend beyond what would be considered usual in adolescence. A recent study by Shaw et al. [15] that included mothers and fathers of adolescents with a range of chronic conditions (asthma, epilepsy and osteogenesis perfecta), showed that parents experience their roles as time-consuming, stressful and unrelenting; but necessary to protect children from harm in the face of multiple risks and uncertainties. This is heightened further where young people have profound and multiple learning difficulties and have a continuing dependency on parents to meet and advocate for them across ecological levels [21–23]. For some parents, transition is also a time where their children may be experiencing deteriorating health due to physical changes [22]. Parents are therefore required to engage in both 'ordinary' parenting that is not directly linked to their child's condition and 'extraordinary' parenting which is specific to their child's healthcare needs [24].

It is important to remember that these parenting demands also exist within a wider context. Parents may have other caring responsibilities (e.g. siblings, partners or ageing parents) and need to maintain relationships with partners, work commitments and engagement in other valued activities. Parents may also have preexisting issues to contend with (e.g. their own health conditions) or be facing major life-events (e.g. divorce, bereavement) that can impact on parenting. It is not surprising, therefore, that some parents describe transition as a 'stressful' and 'difficult process' [4, 15]. Indeed, a number of systematic reviews and meta-analyses have found that parents of children with chronic conditions (including adolescents) report significantly more parenting stress, anxiety, depression and physical health issues than parents of healthy children [25, 26]. Parents also describe how such 'extended' parenting can impact on important aspects of personal development as mid-life adults, making it more challenging to pursue goals relevant to this stage of life (e.g. vocational and financial security, increased opportunities to develop new interests or socialise) [15].

Despite this, the available evidence also suggests that parents value their parenting roles and see them as essential in transition for the immediate and longer-term benefit of their children [4, 15]. A systematic review and thematic synthesis of parenting in transition shows that parents understand the importance of independence-building, as well as young people's acquisition of self-care skills, including disease-management and self-advocacy [4]. It also reveals how parents consciously begin the process of transferring responsibility for managing their condition outside of the clinic context; as part of wider decisions about a young person's developmental readiness and in response to other events in a young person's life (e.g. school residential trips) or family circumstances (e.g. being home alone while parents are working). The timing of this is often based on parental beliefs about a young person's competence and motivation to undertake self-management tasks as well as the stability of the child's condition [4]. Thus, the transfer of responsibility usually occurs incrementally through a 'process of mediated condition management' (p. 82) where parents employ multiple strategies to promote young people's health and development, for example: information-giving, modelling self-care behaviours, prompting, monitoring condition management, allowing young people to experience (non-severe) consequences of their actions [4].

Findings and recommendations from this review certainly support the idea that parents can be key facilitators of their child's transition to adulthood and independent self-management [4, 27], and suggest that parents should be conceived of as assets or resources who can promote the child's adaptation to self-care through a process of family management [28, 29]. This approach is consistent with Social Development Theory [30] which suggests that learning occurs during the interaction between individuals and more knowledgeable others (e.g. parents or health professionals), and that a greater range of skills are developed with adult guidance than would be attained alone. Thus, outcomes for young people are likely to be better when parents are able and willing to support their child's acquisition of skills; moving towards a state of inter-dependence as a bridge to young person independence.

Research is clear on the protective and enabling nature of parental involvement in terms of disease control and reinforces the value of a parent–adolescent partnership in the management of chronic conditions [1, 31–33]. For example, there is now a substantial body of evidence that indicates that compassionate parental involvement can support better glycaemic control in adolescents with diabetes. However, getting the balance right is critical, as research also reveals that parents can experience increased levels of stress and depression that are related to the burden of diabetes management and this negative impact on parents can subsequently place young people at risk of poor outcomes [34–38]. For example, a longitudinal study of parents and young people aged 8–15 years ($n = 174$) with diabetes found almost a third of parents reported low wellbeing which was associated with unsupportive diabetes parenting behaviour, parental distress and behavioural problems in young people, which in turn was linked to reduced glycaemic control [35]. The authors therefore concluded that interventions to help young people manage their condition may also need support for parents.

Thus, it appears that parental involvement in transition can protect young people's health, but may require support to ensure positive outcomes. Research is less clear about how parental involvement fits with increased young person autonomy and other goals in transitional care (e.g. lone consulting). Indeed, there are tensions between the adolescent health literature which emphasises the benefits of independent self-management, and evidence that continued parental involvement contributes to better health outcomes. This tension is mirrored by parents themselves who, on a daily basis, struggle to strike the right balance between protecting young people's health and facilitating their independence [11, 13, 15]. While parents have described wanting to move towards more indirect forms of parenting as their children mature (e.g. through monitoring, teaching self-care skills, guidance and advocacy), they find it difficult to shift from a 'hands on' approach when risks to health are felt to be high or uncertain [15]. This is consistent with some theories about parenting in adolescence, which suggest that parents are driven to protect children's 'physical, psychological, spiritual, ethnic and cultural integrity', but protecting health and survival precedes most other goals ([39], p. 456). From this stance, many parents who at first, appear to be 'over-involved' in young people's care, may be better viewed as following natural parenting imperatives to protect their children from real and anticipated dangers [15].

Health transitions are therefore just one of many overlapping transitions that parents are attempting to navigate and support in adolescence and emerging adulthood. This point has been made by Farre and McDonagh [3] who discuss the 'interrelated nature of health transitions' in detail; explaining how young people undergo multiple transitions (biological, psychological, social, health, educational) which occur alongside, and in connection with one another—with different implications at different developmental stages. However, the way in which parents approach and enact their changing roles has important implications for young people. Indeed, parents' beliefs, expectations and behaviours are known to influence young people's behaviours and subsequent health outcomes [40, 41], and also health professionals' thoughts and behaviours [42]. Understanding how parents can shape young people's outcomes is therefore relevant.

6.2.2 Parenting Capabilities in Transition

New ways of conceptualising parents' roles in transition suggest that a strengths-based approach to parenting is appropriate and needed [43]. This assumes that parents and young people are capable of working together in transition, if they are enabled and supported to do so. The intention is not to ignore or minimise problems, or to set aside young people's safety as the main priority. The focus is, however, on helping parents to use their personal knowledge, skills and potential capabilities to inform positive strategies for transition. Indeed, the literature provides ample evidence that many parents have considerable expertise in their child's condition, are motivated to support their children in transition and have valuable insight into their lives [4]. That said, it is important to recognise that individual capacities can vary considerably, which may cause parenting roles to be expressed in many different ways. As such, parents will differ in their abilities to promote young people's health, wellbeing and transition readiness. Although this has received only limited attention in relation to transitional care [44], evidence from other literatures suggest a number of factors that influence parents' abilities to support young people, including: (a) the personal and psychological functioning of the parent, (b) the characteristics of the young person and (c) the contextual sources of stress and support [39, 45]. Core concepts outlined by these literatures are summarised here, although their implications for practice are revisited later in the chapter.

1. *Personal and psychological functioning of the parent:* In terms of personal and psychological attributes, *connection (or warmth)* is considered to be an important determinant of positive adolescent development, including in families where children/adolescents have a chronic condition [44]. This refers to the emotional closeness of the relationship between parents and their children and constitutes a range of behaviours that parents use to express that young people are loved and accepted. Thus, while an important goal of adolescent development is to form relationships outside of the family, maintaining ongoing connections with parents remains important. Parental *behavioural control* (or regulation, limit-setting) is also important. This involves parents using a range of reasonable techniques to encourage or limit young people's behaviours, in ways that are developmentally appropriate and responsive to their abilities. It includes knowledge and understanding of young people's behaviour, ongoing supervision and monitoring of their activities, communicating clear expectations for behaviour, setting rules and imposing appropriate consequences if these are broken. However, it is also important that parents *respect individuality*; promoting their children's positive self-worth and identity. This involves an appropriate balance of power (where young people can express their opinions, contribute to family decisions, assert their individuality) and the avoidance of psychological control (excessive criticism, invalidating feelings, constraining self-expression, or control through guilt or withdrawal of affection). Parents can also promote better outcomes through *modelling appropriate behaviours*; adopting behaviours and attitudes that are supportive of health and wellbeing, and helping young people

interpret wider social and cultural norms. Although the views of peers begin to have increasing weight, parents still remain an important source of influence for young people. Thus, parents can convey important values through their words and actions. They can also teach young people skills that will support self-management, and increase more generic aspects of their physical safety and psychological wellbeing.

2. *The characteristics of the young person* can also affect parenting, including gender and age, personality and condition. While some of these may remain stable over time, others may change and require new types of parental response. For example, children may develop new symptoms with age or lose abilities as health deteriorates. Recent neurological evidence also reveals that the brain changes more during adolescence than any other time (apart from infancy). These changes also go on for longer than previously thought, with brain 'maturity' not reached until the mid-to-late twenties [46]. However, because changes do not always process smoothly, it is likely that behaviour will be influenced by whichever region is exerting the most power. Thus, there may be times where young people are more vulnerable to the effects of new environmental stresses, are less able to think about the consequences of their actions and have heightened sensitivity to other people's reactions [46–48]. Parenting may be easier when parents have insight into these changes and are able to adapt their approach to ensure a good fit between the young person's characteristics and their own.

3. *Contextual sources of stress and support* are important aspects of parenting in the context of transitional care, but often overlooked. Whatever their circumstances, parents cannot provide all of the support and opportunities that young people require to successfully transition into adulthood. While parents can certainly support their children to access other enabling resources that exist outside of the family (e.g. education, healthcare, formal and informal social networks), other factors can affect their ability to do so. Parenting may be more difficult when there are other caring commitments, physical or mental health issues, lack of financial resources, poor housing, and personal histories that affect caring abilities. It may be difficult for parents to engage in tasks to model and effectively teach self-management strategies when, for example, they are preoccupied with providing basic protections, such as a safe place to live or adequate food.

Many aspects of parenting are therefore amenable to change, for the benefit of parents and young people. This may be particularly important, given evidence that parents who have children and young people with chronic physical conditions may find it harder to adopt positive parenting styles, when compared with parents of healthy children [49]. Helping these parents to recognise and build on their existing strengths within these domains, and foster new parenting skills, will undoubtedly support their ability to promote better outcomes for young people. The Family Management Style Framework [50] offers one such approach. This framework was developed to enhance understanding of how families incorporate the work of managing a child's chronic condition within family life and has provided the conceptual underpinnings for studies of family life in the context of childhood chronic conditions. The framework outlines four major components that can influence family management style and outcomes for individual and family functioning—and which align with the above domains of parenting capacity: (1) contextual influences (social networks, care providers, resources), (2) definition of the situation (child identity, view of the condition, management mindset, parental mutuality), (3) management behaviours (parenting philosophy, management approach) and (4) perceived consequences (family focus, future expectations). Of course, family management changes over the course of a child's life as they mature and develop the skills, cognitive ability and social confidence to manage their own health care activities [28]. However, it is clear that incorporating a flexible approach that supports positive realignment of roles and responsibilities is more consistent with how adults successfully manage their conditions, with support from friends and family. As Morris et al. [51] and others [52, 53] suggest, many of the practices of chronic condition management in adulthood involve the support and/or negotiation of multiple supportive actors and relationships (family focused, friend focused or health care professional focused). This challenges the prevailing notion of 'self'-management as an individual construct and instead highlights the importance of relationships which represent the context in which condition management practices, such as appointment attendance, medication and lifestyle management, are integrated into everyday life.

6.3 Parenting and Transitional Care

6.3.1 Changing Conceptualisations of Parenting in Transitional Care

The World Health Organisation (WHO), in their global overview of adolescent health, states that policies and programmes should 'focus beyond the individual' to improve young people's outcomes [48]. This includes parents and caregivers, who are considered to be major determinants of young people's health, development and wellbeing [48]. Indeed, parents are described as an important protective factor for adolescent health and wellbeing, and as such, the WHO calls for greater understanding and support for positive parenting.

This view has also been expressed in relation to healthcare transition, with several authors emphasising the value of socio-ecological models [54] as a conceptual basis for improved service provision [3, 4, 23, 55–57]. These approaches emphasise how young people with chronic or life-threatening conditions live within the context of their families, peers, social networks, service providers, social values, national policies, laws and resources that interact to influence their health and health-related behaviours. Young people's choices, goals and actions in transition are therefore shaped by a range of actors, relationships and exposures in their immediate and wider environments—not just their own individual characteristics. Healthcare transition can therefore be characterised as a multifaceted process that (at the very least) requires the engagement of patients, families and healthcare providers [55].

Evidence for the appropriateness of this model comes from Schwartz et al. [55, 56] who used stakeholder input to develop and validate the Social-ecological Model of Adolescent and Young Adult Readiness to Transition (SMART). The model contends that transition involves numerous stakeholders (adolescents and young adults, parents, providers), psychological factors that are amenable to change (e.g. self-efficacy) and less modifiable factors (e.g. age, gender, medical status). Further evidence comes from a systematic review that synthesised qualitative findings using an ecological model to understand transition from school to adult services for young people with severe or profound intellectual disability [23].

However, this systemic view has not always been evident in the transitional care literature, where the role of parents has been somewhat marginalised. Until recently, parental inclusion in transition-related research and service development has generally focused on parents' views of the quality of young people's care or providing proxy ratings for young people's outcomes, rather than exploration of parenting roles and needs [4]. Instead, evidence for transition has focused on the perspectives of young patients [58–60], transitional care models [61–63], healthcare practices [21, 64–68] and barriers to transition [19]. Where parents have been considered, their roles in transition care have often been positioned as problematic. This is evident in several systematic reviews of studies across a range of conditions that have identified 'helicopter', 'over-involved' and 'excessive' parenting as a threat to successful transition [19, 69]. Gray et al. [19] suggest that such parenting styles limit young people's opportunities to develop self-management skills and recommend education and guidance for parents. One could argue that such recommendations imply that parents are at fault and their parenting styles require correction. The reality, however, is far more complex. Parents cannot be conceived of as merely observing their child's transition, or as an impediment to it. Rather they are an integral component. They affect the process, and are reciprocally affected by it [55, 56].

This shift in the way parents are constructed in their child's transition is beginning to gain traction. Clinical guidance in the UK, for example, recognises the positive role of parents in managing childhood onset chronic conditions at many levels throughout transition and calls for improved parental support as a key component of transitional care [70]. However, there remains scant advice about what positive parenting looks like and how it can be facilitated in practice. The following sections therefore examine how parents experience current models of transitional care, highlighting areas of inadequacy, and discuss how the conceptualisations of parenting described here offer a useful starting point for service improvement.

6.3.2   Parents Experiences of Transitional Care

While parents are responsible for adapting their role to support their children, healthcare providers are responsible for providing transitional care that addresses the needs of both parents and young people. This is an explicit expectation of policy makers [70, 71] who assert that the active and appropriate involvement of parents in transitional care will lead to better outcomes. This premise has been supported by existing research for some time [6, 72, 73]. More recently, Suris et al. [74] showed that parental satisfaction with their involvement in transitional care was associated with easier transition from the young person's point of view. 'Appropriate parent involvement' was also found to be a feature of transitional care associated with better outcomes in a UK-based longitudinal observational study of 374 young people and their parents/carers across three conditions [75]. Unfortunately, less than half of these participants experienced their transitional care as satisfactory, echoing earlier studies of parental (dis)satisfaction [76]. Others have also found shortfalls between policy and practice with respect to parental involvement and support. A UK report by the Care Quality Commission found that health professionals showed little concern or support for parents in their roles as carers and concluded that there was 'a culture of overreliance on partner agencies to recognise and assess the demands on family members as carers' ([22], p. 11).

Therefore, despite acknowledgement of the need for parent-targeted transition support, this is one aspect of transitional care that remains poorly addressed. Even when available, the provision for parents is often withdrawn at the time they need it most [7]. Parents have described stark contrasts between paediatric and adult care cultures; portraying the journey as one that moves them from care that is tailored to the child's 'unique and complex' needs [77] within a 'warm, familiar, cosy and trusted' environment [78] to a service environment where parents experience 'loss' of support, resources and trusted relationships [79]. As such, the process of transition and the transfer between services have been regarded by parents as a form of 'abandonment and rejection' by paediatric professionals [22, 80], with parents subsequently 'left to get on with it' by adult providers [22].

What is evident, is that parents display extensive knowledge about their children's conditions and play a crucial role in shoring-up current deficiencies in transitional care. A systematic literature review [4] and quality assessment [22] both reveal how parents often act as transition coordinators for their children's care and services; assuming responsibility for communicating between providers; organising orientation visits, clinic appointments at new places of care and transfer of clinical notes. This is even more pronounced in parents whose children have profound and multiple learning difficulties or complex health care needs [22, 23, 81]. Reasons for adopting this role have included: having no lead professional responsible for transition, insufficient service resources and capacity, and fragmented provision. Thus, while parents value the expertise and dedication of their healthcare teams, they perceive transitional care to be complex, confusing and lacking continuity in personnel [4, 15, 22]. They also highlight a lack of joined-up care working within and across sectors, including health, social care and education [4, 15, 22]. To compensate, parents employ a wide range of 'proactive' strategies, including the compilation of hand-held records to document young people's medical histories and service use, and evidence of symptoms and side effects (e.g. video recordings) [15]. Nevertheless, a plethora of parental concerns remain about the current state of transitional care [4, 19, 22] including:

- Lack of information about transition arrangements and the services available to young people and their families
- Loss of long-standing relationships professionals in paediatric care, who provide important support systems for them and their children
- Timing of transfer, which parents prefer to be at times of (relative) stability or wellness
- Developmental readiness of young people, given expectations of reduced parental involvement
- Reduced quality of care in adult services (e.g. beliefs that professionals lack knowledge about conditions with childhood/adolescent onset, reduced time allocated for clinic appointment, loss of specialist services)
- Changes and differences in funding/insurance arrangements and eligibility criteria for medical and social care, services (e.g. respite), specialist equipment and supplies
- Concerns about changes regarding consent and mental capacity
- Lack of parental facilities/involvement (e.g. ability to stay with young person during inpatient admissions)

It is no wonder, therefore, that parents perceive care providers as having insufficient understanding of the impact of transition upon them [22]. It is also unsurprising that they call for rapid improvement including: better collaboration between paediatric and adult sectors; joint visits; starting the process of transition earlier; increased information provision, transition preparation and access to emotional support [4]. These findings and improvement strategies are echoed in many studies [24, 74–76, 82–88] and appear relevant across conditions and countries [4]. The consistency of these findings over the years amply supports the idea that parents are not just integral to the provision of good transitional care, but *need* transitional care themselves.

6.3.3 Parent-Friendly Transitional Care

Although criteria exist to assess youth friendly care [89–92], there are no comparable frameworks to judge the extent to which transitional care is responsive to parental needs. There are however, a number of important concepts that the literature suggests are important.

Models of care provision that recognise parents as determinants of young people's health and wellbeing The models of care in which transitional care services are embedded matter. Existing services may be set up in ways that do not always lend themselves to developmentally appropriate care and appropriate parent involvement. Although 'appropriate parent involvement' has been associated with improved outcomes of transitional care [75], arguably, this is not a feature specific to transitional care, but rather a defining feature of developmentally appropriate healthcare for all young people [93]. Therefore, a model of care rooted in good, routine developmentally appropriate healthcare for all young people should, by definition, incorporate appropriate parent involvement for those requiring transitional care. Concepts that underpin developmentally appropriate care and implications for transitional care practice are discussed further in Chaps. 3 and 8 and by Farre and McDonagh [3].

Valuing parents as assets Healthcare practitioners need to work in partnership with parents in order to help them to facilitate their child's transition and to maintain their own psychological wellbeing during a stage of parenting that is characterised by ambiguity, uncertainty and risk. Importantly, parents need to be acknowledged for all the good work they do and the expertise they bring. They possess unique insights into their child and their condition, in contexts that extend beyond the consultation room. Thus, while transitional care should be centred on young people and promote their own agency, it is also important to view parents as having expertise that can support the individualised nature and practical implementation of transitional care. Working together as a group, where everyone's good intentions are validated, offers opportunities for less adversarial and more constructive approaches in transition. Indeed, integration of young people's perspectives with those of their parents and professionals is a central tenet of family-centred care [94]. Unfortunately, while young people, parents and professionals generally value collaborative practices, in reality, misalignment of expectations and motivations can make this hard to achieve [94]. Indeed, sharing care is often experienced as tensions between parents and young people (e.g. [17]) and parents and professionals [15]. Parents in the same households/families may also have divergent views about the best ways forward [13]. Transitional care that values parents as assets, therefore requires collaborative and compassionate working practices that include: listening to parents, respecting their expertise, acknowledging the stresses and challenges of parenting in transition, supporting unmet needs and integrating parental roles in ways that support young people appropriately [4, 94].

Developmentally appropriate transition plans—for young people and parents The importance of providing a holistic and planned approach to transitional care is well established [95, 96] and assessing the readiness for transfer is a key defining feature of transitional care. In this context, there has been some interest and debate around the use of checklists and measurement tools to assist with this process [97, 98]. However, despite the well documented multi-stakeholder nature of transitional care and multifaceted nature of judging readiness, most tools focus solely on the young person's perception of their own readiness. Only a few tools acknowledge the role and impact of parents on health transition by encompassing parent-reported assessments of their children's readiness or assessments of their own parental readiness. These include some generic tools [97, 99–101] as well as some condition-specific tools [102–104]. These can be excellent conversation starters to assess the understanding and needs of parents in relation to young people's transitional care and prompt appropriate support responses. However, they do not in themselves promote a partnership approach and can become tick-box exercises that inadvertently reinforce the message that parents are a barrier to transitional care. They can also have a narrow focus (i.e. parent understanding and skills in relation to the transition process and self-management), rather than encompassing factors that impact on their experience of transition or parenting capacity. However, when used as part of a well-designed programme, in combination with other initiatives, they can help young people, parents and professionals assess their needs, develop shared expectations, review progress and plan ahead for a range of foreseeable scenarios. Ideally, these should outline and support appropriate parent involvement in relation to all three stages of transition, including the initial preparation phase spanning adolescence, the shorter phase around transfer and the third phase when young people engage with the new adult services [105]. They should be used within a family-centred approach [106] that facilitates dialogue and understanding about what matters to young people and their parents, including their preferences for involvement in transitional care and ambitions for the future. Thus, the focus is not on having a 'one size fits all' model, but on gaining information within a flexible collaborative relationship, to guide the plan (remembering that the checklists are not the plan!).

Supporting parents in relation to young people's rights   Young people have important patient rights in transitional care, including the rights to be seen alone, confidentiality and consent to treatments (where capacity allows). These are a cornerstone of transitional care and key to enabling adolescent autonomy. However, stakeholders' attitudes around this remain controversial and ambivalent, even among parents [87]. Parents have described confusion about changes regarding consent and mental capacity during adolescence, which are not always explained or understood [22]. Adjusting to being excluded from consultations is also a difficult process for parents, particularly when they perceive their child is not coping well [14]. In addition, there is an implicit tension arising from two bodies of evidence that must be carefully balanced in practice; namely the importance and benefits of young people being seen alone [8, 12] versus the protective nature of parental involvement in terms of disease control [1, 31]. Healthcare providers may be able to resolve some of these issues by introducing families to the concept of *inter-dependence* (rather than solely focusing on individual *independence*) and supporting them to practice a partnership approach which incrementally engages the young person in developmentally appropriate self-care and advocacy. In terms of lone consultations, one could argue that most adult patients are afforded the right to attend consultations with family members or other trusted individuals. Young people should certainly have opportunities to be seen alone and given support to instigate this safely and without negative repercussions (given the power imbalances that usually exists in relation to young people and their parents). However, the focus should not be on insisting that young person are seen alone, unless there are very good reasons for this. Instead, health professionals need to ensure that both young people and parents understand their rights as patients and carers, and that young people have opportunities to develop and practice self-advocacy skills, make informed decisions about who is involved in their care (including consultations) and have support to access to specialist services (e.g. patient advocacy services, family mediating services).

Further research on how to effectively balance these two sets of recommendations is still needed [31], with greater consideration of these ethical aspects of transitional care [107]. In the meantime, there is the potential for better addressing the journey towards young people's independence without undermining parental involvement by starting preparation for transition early on in adolescence [78]. Alongside this, current best practice guidelines also emphasise the need to regularly discuss with young people how they would like their parents to be involved throughout their transition [70].

Support to manage risk, uncertainty and vulnerability An important component of effective transitional care is supporting families to cope with risk and uncertainty. Indeed, parents who face higher levels of illness-related uncertainty are likely to perceive their child as vulnerable [108] and engage in and more activities to protect their children from harm [15, 109, 110]). It was shown earlier in this chapter that parents often want to foster increased independence in their children, but struggle to transfer responsibilities when they perceive that the risks to health are high or uncertain. While this can have a protective function for their health, there are also important reasons why families should be supported to manage risk and uncertainty. These additional care-giving demands can negatively impact on parents' wellbeing, which further reduces their capacity to promote young people's development and wellbeing [34–38, 109, 110]. Research also suggests that parents' strategies to manage uncertainty can be counterproductive by exacerbating uncertainty, diminishing hope or increasing distress [15, 111]. For example, constant monitoring of young people's health can highlight symptoms and signs that parents are unsure how to respond to, causing additional anxiety and straining relationships as young people become frustrated with parental surveillance [15]. Health professionals therefore need to provide regular opportunities for parents and young people to discuss issues around risk, uncertainty and vulnerability, and work collaboratively to prioritise their concerns and make developmentally appropriately plans to manage anticipated scenarios. Existing frameworks (e.g. [112]) may help them to understand the different types of uncertainty that might be relevant to families. This may involve addressing uncertainties related to the young person's condition, generic adolescent health and wellbeing issues, role of parents in transition, and the organisation of services [15]. A positive youth development approach [113] (Chap. 2) may be particularly beneficial by demonstrating that young people have the potential to manage risk and explaining how parents and other people (including care providers) can support them to achieve this. A promising resource in relation to this is The Skills for Growing Up (SGU) communication tool (Chap. 8), which aims to promote autonomy and empowerment for young people in hospital or rehabilitation care [114–116]. This is age appropriate, covers a broad range of aspects of daily life and is underpinned by a shared management approach where young people and their parents work together to identify and set goals [114–116]. Importantly, the SGU is considered relevant to conditions where managing risk is a core concern for parents, including epilepsy [115]. The focus is not on avoiding all risks, but developing the knowledge, skills and confidence that allow young people to recognise and prepare for risk, including insight about when to act for themselves and when to seek help. This is likely to require (1) the identification of different risks, (2) awareness of how these affect young people, parents and others around them, (3) understanding the benefits of addressing risks, including the reduction of harm, personal growth, increased opportunities and reduced parental stress, (4) support to develop self-management skills and (5) the provision of 'safe' opportunities to experience manageable levels of risk and responsibility in ways that are demonstrable to parents. Healthcare providers could encourage problem solving in clinics, offer skills workshops, signpost wider opportunities (e.g. those offered by charities/youth organisations), and encourage families to create opportunities at home for their children to learn and practice skills. This will be an essential part of a young person's transitional readiness, which is an important predictor of successful transition to adult healthcare [33, 117].

Support for parenting capacity Despite acknowledgement that transition impacts on parental health, wellbeing and development, and evidence that positive parenting can promote better outcomes for young people, transitional care services rarely include processes to assess or address parental support needs [22]. Even when parents' needs are assessed, it can feel like a 'tick-box exercise' [22], particularly when focused narrowly (e.g. on disease education) rather than a more holistic assessment of their wider emotional and practical needs. However, it is also evident that many professionals have no training in assessing the needs of parents and lack the resources to address any needs identified [22]. Unfortunately, intervention studies specific to parenting and transition remain limited. Most research has focused on interventions to improve parental management of treatments [44]. There are, however, some limited systematic and scoping reviews that have examined psychological interventions for parents of children and adolescents with chronic illness [118] and medical complexity [119]. These have examined the effect of a range of therapies (e.g. cognitive-behavioural therapy, family therapy, motivational interviewing and problem-solving therapy) on parents' physical and mental health, parenting skills and behaviour. The findings are not easy to apply, as the results pertaining to parents of adolescents cannot be separated from that of younger patients. In general, the findings suggest that *some* parents can experience modest benefits from interventions, but the heterogeneity of the data and other design limitations (such as explicit criteria about the goodness of fit between parents' needs and interventions) makes it difficult to draw firm conclusions. However, Bradshaw et al. [119] conclude that the results confirm that parents have 'significant and diverse support needs, and are likely to benefit from a number of interventions targeting specific issues and outcomes across their child's condition trajectory'. Less attention has been placed on parenting styles and behaviours. Johnson et al. [120] have highlighted the need for effective family therapy interventions, especially those addressing parenting in healthcare settings.

Parents themselves have often called for more opportunities for parent-to-parent support during transition; the potential of which has been suggested for some time across different types of support and conditions [15, 121–127]. Networking support typically includes peer support groups, parent-led transition groups, befriending, internet support groups, and lay-led or specialist workshops. Recent studies show that such initiatives can be an important source of hope, motivation and connection to resources for parents during transition, particularly as they offer opportunities for shared experience; a critical element of support that health care providers often lack [85]. Reported benefits include new knowledge, becoming more future-oriented, being more active in their transition preparations, decreased feelings of isolation, opportunities to discuss nonclinical issues [123, 128–130]. It also appears that supporting others can be as beneficial as receiving support, enabling parent mentors or befrienders to recognise how much they have developed since their child's diagnosis [131, 132]. However, the benefits are less substantiated in a review of quantitative research studies [126]. Thus, while interventions in this area have shown promise, further research is needed to find effective ways to help parents and young people shift their roles and responsibilities [1] and cope with the impact of transition.

6.4   Key Recommendations for Practice

This chapter provides strong evidence that young people's outcomes are likely to improve if transitional care also includes a focus on parent outcomes. This includes their physical and mental health, and parenting capacity. The evidence also points to the relevance of a strength (or empowerment) based approach which 'explores, in a collaborative way the entire individual's abilities and their circumstances rather than making the deficit the focus of the intervention' ([43], p. 24). As such, transitional care should be based on a holistic picture of young peoples' lives and work with others who are likely to shape their outcomes, including parents and other key people/organisations in their networks such as siblings, teachers and social workers. This approach aligns closely with the theoretical frameworks highlighted previously in the chapter as relevant to transition, including the ecological, developmental, positive youth development, positive parenting and family management models. Existing evidence and theory thus supports the notion that transitional care needs to look beyond the individual patient to optimise their outcomes.

In line with this approach, transitional care providers will need to identify both the strengths and difficulties within the family by undertaking holistic assessments. This should explore the young person's development, the parents' capacity to meet their child's needs, and the impact of wider contextual factors. Although these approaches are more established in social work and mental health provision, they are explicitly relevant to families [133] and are beginning to gain traction in health care. For example, the UK Department for Health and Social Care [43] has developed a framework and handbook to support practitioners understand strengths-based interventions and implement them in practice, including case studies that focus on families and transition to adulthood. The handbook also includes helpful practitioner reflections that explain the rationale, application and benefits of using a strengths-based approach. In terms of parent involvement, this approach goes beyond the assessment and support of skills related to the transfer of self-management skills, but extends more widely to support general parenting capacity. In reality, no single agency is likely to provide all the help that will be required (e.g. addressing barriers related to poverty). However, health professionals, in partnership with families and other agencies, can support parents to develop the skills and resources to begin to address these issues and judge what services and interventions may be relevant.

Providers of health and social care also need to adopt a life-course approach to adolescent health [47]. Not only does this suggest that interventions in adolescence will support better outcomes in adulthood, but also acknowledges that positive or harmful parenting begins long before adolescence [48]. While discussion of this is beyond the scope of this chapter, it is important to recognise that early support for parents will benefit families in transition. Therefore, in addition to improved collaborative working between adolescent and adult care providers, it will also be important to collaborate with early year providers to ensure that parents, whose children are diagnosed with a chronic condition in childhood, have access to parenting support as early as possible. Early year providers can also inform transition planning by communicating important information about specific family needs as part of any their handover to adolescent services. This may not remove all challenges associated with adolescence and transition. However, parenting support received pre-transition and awareness of their ongoing needs may support better outcomes; by equipping parents with the skills to anticipate their children's needs and respond appropriately.

Ensuring dedicated time and effort to supporting parenting capacity will be particularly important. We have already identified some key targets that are amenable to change and offer some practical strategies in Table 6.1. This is not to ignore the limitations of insufficient healthcare funding that can constrain new or extended work. However, there is much that can be done to support parents within existing resources, referral routes and community level networks. Much of this is about cultural changes that require people to think and behave differently. It will require new conversations with young people and their parents such as: What does a good life look like for you and your family? What do you enjoy doing? What level of independence would you/your child like to have? What can you manage now? What would you like to manage soon? In your opinion, what might work better? What support do you need? How can we help?—followed by meaningful action (e.g. [43]). Practical guidance to explore individual's needs, aspirations and capacities have been developed (e.g. [43]) and include examples of strength-based questioning that may be of value to health professionals involved in transitional care.

Realising these ambitions is likely to require new research, interventions and initiatives. It will be important to embed these within coproduction models of involvement [138] to ensure that parents, young people and professionals are equal partners in decision-making. Indeed, it is evident that parents have been largely marginalised in the development of transitional care and rarely involved in developing interventions designed to meet their needs, which may account for the slow progress in finding effective approaches [119]. Yet, there is considerable evidence that young people and their parents are able and willing to comment on their care and services, given the opportunity (e.g. [4, 22]). One mechanism to improve service provision may be through 'learning collaboratives' where professionals and families work together for set periods of time to learn about, coproduce and try new processes. Guidelines to support such approaches in health care are available and are easily transferable to transitional care [139]. Targets for further research and service development, based on this Chapter, are likely to include how to: assess parental capacity and support needs; target interventions to parents/young people at

Table 6.1 Practical suggestions to improve parenting capacity

Personal needs of parents

• Address the developmental changes of mid-life adults and explore how these changes impact on their parenting abilities and relationship with their child. Help them to identify personal goals in transition (e.g. increased independence in young people not only benefit their children but may also mean more time for them to persue valued activities, such as hobbies, or improve opportunities for employment). Where possible, link these opportunities to wider benefits for them, their children and families. Help them to access relevant support (e.g. career guidance).

• Distinguish between parents who normally cope well, but are overwhelmed with specific problems, and those who have more complex or deep-seated needs (e.g. mental health problems or learning disabilities) and may need referral to specialists or multi-agency input (e.g. counselling, community drug and alcohol services).

Parenting capacity

• **Connection:** Provide parents with advice and practical strategies to improve communication with their children that focus on warmth and respect for individuality, including understanding adolescent communication styles, managing arguments and conflict. Provide opportunities for young people and parents to work together on goal setting and help them to celebrate as they move towards their goals.

• **Support for behaviour control:** Help parents to promote positive adolescent behaviour using strategies that recognise their increasing needs for autonomy and privacy. Help them to: establish rules that are specific to young people's condition and related to wider aspects of adolescent health and wellbeing; communicate expectations, limits and reasonable consequences; and strategies to effectively monitor behaviours. Provide specific information that explains how their child's condition and development may reciprocally affect one another. Also provide information about normal adolescent development (e.g. teen brain, sexual health), including stressors associated with this period and symptoms of important adolescent problems (e.g. self-harm, anxiety, depression, eating disorders, bullying, substance abuse). Show parents how to teach important protective skills (e.g. self-care, dealing with peer pressure). Support parents to respond appropriately to their children's emotions and behaviour (e.g. anger, anxiety) and their own feelings in response to these (including where to seek help for them and their children). Facilitate the development of parental networks to help parents learn about and establish positive social/cultural norms.

• **Respect for individuality:** Help parents and young people to gain/maintain mutual respect by acknowledging each other's knowledge, abilities and good intentions, but also their concerns, fears and vulnerabilities. Help parents understand their rights and responsibility to advocate for their children, and children's own rights as patients/young people. Teach parents the skills and knowledge necessary for advocacy, helping them to model these. Help parents to shift from being the main source of information to helping their children find these resources on their own.

Table 6.1 (continued)

• **Modelling appropriate behaviours:** Encourage parents to adopt attitudes and behaviours that support health and wellbeing (e.g. non-smoking, clinic attendance), noting that that young people are also able to spot inconsistencies between what parents say and do! Support them to be a confident and direct source of information (adolescent health and condition specific). Expose parents and young people to other positive role models. Provide opportunities for parents to learn and practice guidance competencies. Strategies to prepare young people for assuming healthcare autonomy might include: parents encouraging, supporting and allowing their child to experience self-care [134]; modelling self-care behaviours, monitoring condition management and prompting treatment administration; actively teaching their children self-management skills, including condition and treatment management, self-advocacy and "self-surveillance" of symptoms [135]; ensuring awareness/access to their own medical history and practicing asking questions for consultations; active provision of practical support with key tasks such as filling prescriptions, making appointments or commuting with clinics [136]. Support young people to plan for/achieve goals beyond their health (e.g. introduction to career counsellors, volunteering).

Contextual sources of stress and support

Assess and address material and financial resources that can impact on parenting capacity (e.g. by actively facilitating access to advice and state/community level programmes that will help parents find the resources they need to adequately support their children). Facilitate care close to home where possible and schedule clinics/programmes/interventions at convenient times, considering access to transportation and costs. Explore and address the impact of family structure and dynamics (e.g. challenges associated with being a single-parent, caring for siblings/aging parents, shared care between parents in two households). Provide parents with opportunities to meet, talk with, and develop meaningful relationships with other parents of adolescents e.g. parent support groups, community parenting programmes, befriending schemes, parenting helplines, safe social media forums. Interventions that support young people are likely to reduce the stress that parents experience e.g. young person support groups, community youth groups, self-management workshops, befriending groups.

Organisational barriers

Minimise sources of uncertainty for parents by providing consistent care (seeing same professionals), joining-up services (within and between health, social and education agencies), continuity at transfer, and transfer at times of health stability. Support families to understand how services are organised, how to access them and strategies for healthcare use and help-seeking. Self-assessment and benchmarking tools to support organisations assess their own practice in transitional care are available (e.g. [70, 137]). However, developing a competent workforce will be important. Many professionals lack training to assess and support the needs of parents [22]. Professionals may benefit from training about family dynamics and how to create safe environments for young people and their parents to discuss and agree transition goals. This should include communication training to support discussions about sensitive/challenging issues and to avoid/resolve conflicts. When discussing transition, staff also need to promote and model positive norms, decision-making and collaborative practices (e.g. listening, respect, compromise). Wider initiatives to promote public understanding of chronic conditions in adolescence are also needed.

most risk and promote optimal benefit; improve workforce competency and collaboration. Attempts to address these will also benefit from using frameworks that support robust design, implementation and evaluation (e.g. [140–143]) to ensure they target parents appropriately, align to outcomes that matter to families and provide optimal benefits.

6.5   Conclusion

In this chapter, we have shown that there has been a discernible shift in our understanding of transitional care, highlighting it as a process that involves young people and their parents who reciprocally shape the experience of transition and influence outcomes. It thus repositions parents as key enablers in transition and protective factors in young people's health and wellbeing, rather than barriers to young person autonomy, as traditionally conceived. We argue that taking a family-focused approach, that recognises the strengths and potential of young people and their parents, is more conceptually appropriate and more likely to bring about better outcomes for all involved. In line with this, we have suggested a number of general principles and practical strategies to help care providers align their practices to models of transitional care policies that recognise parents as major determinants in adolescent health. Such approaches are likely to promote the positive involvement of parents in transitional care and help young people to flourish in transition. It may also address the dissatisfaction that parents and young people express in relation to their care, and explain why even structured programmes often fail to deliver their promised benefits.

References

1. Reed-Knight B, Blount RL, Gilleland J. The transition of health care responsibility from parents to youth diagnosed with chronic illness: a developmental systems perspective. Fam Syst Health. 2014;32(2):219–34. https://doi.org/10.1037/fsh0000039.
2. Coyne I, Sheehan A, Heery E, While AE. Improving transition to adult healthcare for young people with cystic fibrosis: a systematic review. J Child Health Care. 2017;21(3):312–30. https://doi.org/10.1177/1367493517712479.
3. Farre A, McDonagh JE. Helping health services to meet the needs of young people with chronic conditions: towards a developmental model for transition. Healthcare. 2017;5(4):77. https://doi.org/10.3390/healthcare5040077.
4. Heath G, Farre A, Shaw K. Parenting a child with chronic illness as they transition into adulthood: a systematic review and thematic synthesis of parents' experiences. Patient Educ Couns. 2017;100(1):76–92. https://doi.org/10.1016/j.pec.2016.08.011.
5. Kieckhefer GM, Trahms CM, Churchill SS, Simpson JN. Measuring parent-child shared management of chronic illness. Pediatr Nurs. 2009;35(2):101–8.
6. Williams B, Mukhopadhyay S, Dowell J, Coyle J. From child to adult: an exploration of shifting family roles and responsibilities in managing physiotherapy for cystic fibrosis. Soc Sci Med. 2007;65(10):2135–46. https://doi.org/10.1016/j.socscimed.2007.07.020.
7. Allen D, Channon S, Lowes L, Atwell C, Lane C. Behind the scenes: the changing roles of parents in the transition from child to adult diabetes service. Diabet Med. 2011;28(8):994–1000. https://doi.org/10.1111/j.1464-5491.2011.03310.x.
8. Duncan RE, Vandeleur M, Derks A, Sawyer S. Confidentiality with adolescents in the medical setting: what do parents think? J Adolesc Health. 2011;49(4):428–30. https://doi.org/10.1016/j.jadohealth.2011.02.006.
9. Iles N, Lowton K. What is the perceived nature of parental care and support for young people with cystic fibrosis as they enter adult health services? Health Soc Care Commun. 2010;18(1):21–9. https://doi.org/10.1111/j.1365-2524.2009.00871.x.

10. Ivey JB, Wright A, Dashiff CJ. Finding the balance: adolescents with type 1 diabetes and their parents. J Pediatr Health Care. 2009;23:10–8. https://doi.org/10.1016/j.pedhc.2007.12.008.
11. Kleop M, Hendry LB. Letting go or holding on? Parents' perceptions of their relationships with their children during emerging adulthood. Br J Dev Psychol. 2010;28(4):817–34. https://doi.org/10.1348/026151009X480581.
12. Sasse RA, Aroni RA, Sawyer SM, Duncan RE. Confidential consultations with adolescents: an exploration of Australian parents' perspectives. J Adolesc Health. 2013;52(6):786–91. https://doi.org/10.1016/j.jadohealth.2012.11.019.
13. Akré C, Surís J-C. From controlling to letting go: what are the psychosocial needs of parents of adolescents with a chronic illness? Health Educ Res. 2014;29(5):764–72. https://doi.org/10.1093/her/cyu040.
14. Gannoni AF, Shute RH. Parental and child perspectives on adaptation to childhood chronic illness: a qualitative study. Clin Child Psychol Psychiatry. 2010;15(1):39–53. https://doi.org/10.1177/1359104509338432.
15. Shaw K, Baldwin L, Heath G. "A confident parent breeds a confident child." Understanding the experience and needs of parents whose children will transition from paediatric to adult care. J Child Health. 2020; https://doi.org/10.1177/1367493520936422.
16. Arnett JJ. Emerging adulthood: a theory of development from the late teens through the twenties. Am Psychol. 2000;55(5):469–80. https://doi.org/10.1037/0003-066X.55.5.469.
17. Peeters MAC, Hilberink SR, van Staa AL. The road to independence: Lived experiences of youth with chronic conditions and their parents compared. J Pediatr Rehabil Med. 2014;7(1):33–42. https://doi.org/10.3233/PRM-140272.
18. Tierney S, Deaton C, Jones A, Oxley H, Biesty J, Kirk S. Liminality and transfer to adult services: a qualitative investigation involving young people with cystic fibrosis. Int J Nurs Stud. 2013;50(6):738–46. https://doi.org/10.1016/j.ijnurstu.2012.04.014.
19. Gray WN, Schaefer MR, Resmini-Rawlinson A, Wagoner ST. Barriers to transition from pediatric to adult care: a systematic review. J Pediatr Psychol. 2018;43(5):488–502. https://doi.org/10.1093/jpepsy/jsx142.
20. Woodgate RL, Edwards M, Ripat JD, Borton B, Rempel G. Intense parenting: a qualitative study detailing the experiences of parenting children with complex care needs. BMC Pediatr. 2015;15:97. https://doi.org/10.1186/s12887-015-0514-5.
21. Brown M, Macarthur J, Higgins A, Chouliara Z. Transitions from child to adult health care for young people with intellectual disabilities: a systematic review. J Adv Nurs. 2019;75(ii):2418–34. https://doi.org/10.1111/jan.13985.
22. Care Quality Commission (CQC). From the pond into the sea. Children's transition to adult health services. London: CQC; 2014.
23. Jacobs P, MacMahon K, Quayle E. Transition from school to adult services for young people with severe or profound intellectual disability: A systematic review utilizing framework synthesis. J Appl Res Intellect Disabil. 2018;31(6):962–82. https://doi.org/10.1111/jar.12466.
24. Crawford K, Wilson C, Low JK, Manias E, Williams A. Transitioning adolescents to adult nephrology care: a systematic review of the experiences of adolescents, parents, and health professionals. Pediatr Nephrol. 2020;35(4):555–67. https://doi.org/10.1007/s00467-019-04223-9.
25. Cohn LN, Pechlivanoglou P, Lee Y, Mahant S, Orkin J, Marson A, Cohen E. Health outcomes of parents of children with chronic illness: a systematic review and meta-analysis. J Pediatr. 2020;218:166–177.e2. https://doi.org/10.1016/j.jpeds.2019.10.068.
26. Cousino MK, Hazen RA. Parenting stress among caregivers of children with chronic illness: a systematic review. J Pediatr Psychol. 2013;38(8):809–28. https://doi.org/10.1093/jpepsy/jst049.
27. Tuchman LK, Slap GB, Britto MT. Transition to adult care: experiences and expectations of adolescents with a chronic illness. Child Care Health Dev. 2008;34(5):557–63. https://doi.org/10.1111/j.1365-2214.2008.00844.x.

28. Beacham BL, Deatrick JA. Health care autonomy in children with chronic conditions: implications for self-care and family management. Nurs Clin North Am. 2013;48(2):305–17. https://doi.org/10.1016/j.cnur.2013.01.010.
29. Compas BE, Jaser SS, Dunn MJ, Rodriguez EM. Coping with chronic illness in childhood and adolescence. Annu Rev Clin Psychol. 2012;8:455–80. https://doi.org/10.1146/annurev-clinpsy-032511-143108.
30. Vygotsky L. Mind in society: the development of higher psychological processes. Cambridge, MA: Harvard University Press; 1978.
31. Duncan RE, Jekel M, O'Connell MA, Sanci LA, Sawyer SM. Balancing parental involvement with adolescent friendly health care in teenagers with diabetes: are we getting it right? J Adolesc Health. 2014;55(1):59–64. https://doi.org/10.1016/j.jadohealth.2013.11.024.
32. Modi AC, Pai AL, Hommel KA, Hood KK, Cortina S, Hilliard ME, Guilfoyle SM, Gray WN, Drotar D. Pediatric self-management: a framework for research, practice, and policy. Pediatrics. 2012;129(2):e473–85. https://doi.org/10.1542/peds.2011-1635.
33. Wiebe DJ, Chow CM, Palmer DL, Butner J, Butler JM, Osborn P, Berg CA. Developmental processes associated with longitudinal declines in parental responsibility and adherence to type 1 diabetes management across adolescence. J Pediatr Psychol. 2014;39(5):532–41. https://doi.org/10.1093/jpepsy/jsu006.
34. Cunningham RS, Vesco AT, Dolan LM, Hood KK. From caregiver psychological distress to adolescent glycemic control: the mediating role of perceived burden around diabetes management. J Pediatr Psychol. 2011;36(2):196–205. https://doi.org/10.1093/jpepsy/jsq071.
35. Eilander MMA, Snoek FJ, Rotteveel J, Aanstoot HJ, Bakker-van Waarde WM, Houdijk ECAM, Nuboer R, Winterdijk P, de Wit M. Parental diabetes behaviors and distress are related to glycemic control in youth with type 1 diabetes: longitudinal data from the DINO study. J Diabetes Res. 2017;2017:1462064. https://doi.org/10.1155/2017/1462064.
36. Maas-van Schaaijk N, Roeleveld-Versteegh A, van Baar A. The interrelationships among paternal and maternal parenting stress, metabolic control, and depressive symptoms in adolescents with type 1 diabetes mellitus. J Pediatr Psychol. 2013;38(1):30–40. https://doi.org/10.1093/jpepsy/jss096.
37. Mackey E, Struemph K, Powell P, Chen R, Streissand R, Holmes C. Maternal depressive symptoms and disease care status in youth with type 1 diabetes. Health Psychol. 2014;33(8):783–91. https://doi.org/10.1037/hea0000066.
38. Rumburg TM, Lord JH, Savin KL, Jaser SS. Maternal diabetes distress is linked to maternal depressive symptoms and adolescents' glycemic control. Pediatr Diabetes. 2017;18(1):67–70. https://doi.org/10.1111/pedi.12350.
39. Small SA, Eastman G. Rearing adolescents in contemporary society: a conceptual framework for understanding the responsibilities and needs of parents. Fam Relat. 1991;40(4):455–62. https://doi.org/10.2307/584904.
40. Clarizia NA, Chahal N, Manlhiot C, Kilburn J, Redington AN, McCrindle BW. Transition to adult health care for adolescents and young adults with congenital heart disease: perspectives of the patient, parent and health care provider. Can J Cardiol. 2009;25(9):317–22. https://doi.org/10.1016/S0828-282X(09)70145-X.
41. Logan DE, Scharff L. Relationships between family and parent characteristics and functional abilities in children with recurrent pain syndromes: an investigation of moderating effects on the pathway from pain to disability. J Pediatr Psychol. 2005;30(8):698–707. https://doi.org/10.1093/jpepsy/jsj060.
42. Dupuis F, Duhamel F, Gendron S. Transitioning care of an adolescent with cystic fibrosis: development of systemic hypothesis between parents, adolescents, and health care professionals. J Fam Nurs. 2011;17(3):291–311. https://doi.org/10.1177/1074840711414907.
43. Department of Health and Social Care. Strengths-based approach: practice framework and practice handbook. London: Department for Health and Social Care; 2019.
44. Crandell JL, Sandelowski M, Leeman J, Havill NL, Knafl K. Parenting behaviors and the well-being of children with a chronic physical condition. Fam Syst Health. 2018;36(1):45–61. https://doi.org/10.1037/fsh0000305.

45. World Health Organisation. Helping parents in developing countries improve adolescents' health. Geneva: WHO; 2007. https://www.who.int/maternal_child_adolescent/documents/9789241595841/en/.
46. Johnson S, Blum RW, Giedd JN. Adolescent maturity and the brain: the promise and pitfalls of neuroscience research in adolescent health policy. J Adolesc Health. 2010;45(3):216–21. https://doi.org/10.1016/j.jadohealth.2009.05.016.
47. Coleman JC. The nature of adolescence (adolescence and society). 4th ed. London: Routledge; 2011.
48. World Health Organisation. Health for the world's adolescents. A second chance in the second decade. Geneva: WHO; 2014. https://apps.who.int/adolescent/second-decade/.
49. Pinquart M. Do the parent-child relationship and parenting behaviors differ between families with a child with and without chronic illness? A meta-analysis. J Pediatr Psychol. 2013;38(7):708–21. https://doi.org/10.1093/jpepsy/jst020.
50. Knafl KA, Deatrick JA, Havill NL. Continued development of the family management style framework. J Fam Nurs. 2012;18(1):11–34. https://doi.org/10.1177/1074840711427294.
51. Morris RL, Kennedy A, Sanders C. Evolving 'self'-management: exploring the role of social network typologies on individual long-term condition management. Health Expect. 2015;19(5):1044–61. https://doi.org/10.1111/hex.12394.
52. Dwarswaard J, Bakker EJ, van Staa A, Boeije HR. Self-management support from the perspective of patients with a chronic condition: a thematic synthesis of qualitative studies. Health Expect. 2016;19(2):194–208. https://doi.org/10.1111/hex.12346.
53. Gallant MP. The influence of social support on chronic illness self-management: a review and directions for research. Health Educ Behav. 2003;30(2):170–95. https://doi.org/10.1177/1090198102251030.
54. Bronfenbrenner U, Morris PA. The ecology of developmental processes. In: Damon W, Lerner RM, editors. Handbook of child psychology: theoretical models of human development. Hoboken, NJ: John Wiley & Sons Inc.; 1998. p. 993–1028.
55. Schwartz LA, Tuchman LK, Hobbie WL, Ginsberg JP. A social-ecological model of readiness for transition to adult-oriented care for adolescents and young adults with chronic health conditions. Child Care Health Dev. 2011;37(6):883–95. https://doi.org/10.1111/j.1365-2214.2011.01282.
56. Schwartz LA, Brumley LD, Tuchman LK, Barakat LP, Hobbie WL, Ginsberg JP, Daniel LC, Kazak AE, Bevans K, Deatrick JA. Stakeholder validation of a model of readiness for transition to adult care. JAMA Pediatr. 2013;167(10):939–46. https://doi.org/10.1001/jamapediatrics.2013.2223.
57. Wang G, McGrath BB, Watts C. Health care transitions among youth with disabilities or special health care needs: an ecological approach. J Pediatr Nurs. 2010;25(6):505–50. https://doi.org/10.1016/j.pedn.2009.07.003.
58. Betz CL, Lobo ML, Nehring WM, Bui K. Voices not heard: a systematic review of adolescents' and emerging adults' perspectives of health care transition. Nurs Outlook. 2013;61(5):311–36. https://doi.org/10.1016/j.outlook.2013.01.008.
59. Fegran L, Hall EO, Uhrenfeldt L, Aagaard H, Ludvigsen MS. Adolescents' and young adults' transition experiences when transferring from paediatric to adult care: a qualitative metasynthesis. Int J Nurs Stud. 2014;51(1):123–35. https://doi.org/10.1016/j.ijnurstu.2013.02.001.
60. Lugasi T, Achille M. Stevenson Patients' Perspective on factors that facilitate transition from child-centered to adult-centered health care: a theory integrated meta-summary of quantitative and qualitative studies. J Adolesc Health. 2011;48(5):429–40. https://doi.org/10.1016/j.jadohealth.2010.10.016.
61. Betz CL. Different healthcare transition models. In: Hergenroeder A, Wiemann CM, editors. Health care transition. Cham: Springer; 2018. p. 363–77. ISBN: 978-3-319-72867-4.
62. Kime N., Bagnall AM, Day R. Systematic review of transition models for young people with long-term conditions: a report for NHS diabetes. 2013. http://eprints.leedsbeckett.ac.uk/606/.

63. Watson R, Parr JR, Joyce C, May C, Le Couteur AS. Models of transitional care for young people with complex health needs: a scoping review. Child Care Health Dev. 2011;37(6):780–91. https://doi.org/10.1111/j.1365-2214.2011.01293.

64. Bhawra J, Toulany A, Cohen E, Moore Hepburn C, Guttmann A. Primary care interventions to improve transition of youth with chronic health conditions from paediatric to adult healthcare: a systematic review. BMJ Open. 2016;6:e011871. https://doi.org/10.1136/bmjopen-2016-011871.

65. Campbell F, Biggs K, Aldiss SK, O'Neill PM, Clowes M, McDonagh J, While A, Gibson F. Transition of care for adolescents from paediatric services to adult health services. Cochrane Database Syst Rev. 2016;4:CD009794. https://doi.org/10.1002/14651858.CD009794.pub2.

66. Chu P, Maslow G, von Isenburg M, Chung R. Systematic review of the impact of transition interventions for adolescents with chronic illness on transfer from pediatric to adult healthcare. J Pediatr Nurs. 2015;30:e19–27. https://doi.org/10.1016/j.pedn.2015.05.022.

67. Crowley R, Wolfe I, Lock K, McKee M. Improving the transition between paediatric and adult healthcare: a systematic review. Arch Dis Child. 2011;96(6):548–53. https://doi.org/10.1136/adc.2010.202473.

68. While A, Forbes A, Ullman R, Lewis S, Mathes L, Griffiths P. Good practices that address continuity during transition from child to adult care: synthesis of the evidence. Child Care Health Dev. 2004;30(5):439–52. https://doi.org/10.1111/j.1365-2214.2004.00440.

69. Nehring WM, Betz CL, Lobo ML. Uncharted territory: systematic review of providers' roles, understanding, and views pertaining to health care transition. J Pediatr Nurs. 2015;30(5):732–47. https://doi.org/10.1016/j.pedn.2015.05.030.

70. National Institute for Health and Care Excellence (NICE). NICE guidelines [NG43] Transition from children's to adults' services for young people using health or social care services. 2016. https://www.nice.org.uk/guidance/ng43.

71. Canadian Association of Pediatric Health Centres (CAPHC), National Transitions Community of Practice. (2016). A guideline for transition from paediatric to adult health care for youth with special health care needs: a national approach.

72. Geerts E, van de Wiel H, Tamminga R. A pilot study on the effects of the transition of paediatric to adult health care in patients with haemophilia and in their parents: patient and parent worries, parental illness-related distress and health-related quality of life. Haemophilia. 2008;14(5):1007–13. https://doi.org/10.1111/j.1365-2516.2008.01798.x.

73. Meah A, Callery P, Milnes L, Rogers S. Thinking 'taller': sharing responsibility in the everyday lives of children with asthma. J Clin Nurs. 2010;19(13–14):1952–9. https://doi.org/10.1111/j.1365-2702.2008.02767.x.

74. Suris JC, Larbre J-P, Hofer M, Hauschild M, Barrense-Dias Y, Berchtold A, Akre C. Transition from paediatric to adult care: what makes it easier for parents? Child Care Health Dev. 2017;43(1):152–5. https://doi.org/10.1016/j.pedn.2019.03.016.

75. Colver A, McConachie H, Le Couteur A, Dovey-Pearce G, Mann KD, McDonagh JE, Pearce MS, Vale L, Merrick H, Parr JR, Bennett C, Maniatopoulos G, Rapley T, Reape D, Chater N, Gleeson H, Billson A, Bem A, Bennett S, On behalf of the Transition Collaborative Group. A longitudinal, observational study of the features of transitional healthcare associated with better outcomes for young people with long-term conditions. BMC Med. 2018;16(1):111. https://doi.org/10.1186/s12916-018-1102-y.

76. Sonneveld HM, Strating MMH, van Staa AL, Nieboer AP. Gaps in transitional care: what are the perceptions of adolescents, parents and providers? Transitional care - perceptions of adolescents, parents and providers. Child Care Health Dev. 2013;39(1):69–80. https://doi.org/10.1111/j.1365-2214.2011.01354.x.

77. Davies H, Rennick J, Majnemer A. Transition from pediatric to adult health care for young adults with neurological disorders: parental perspectives. Can J Neurosci Nurs. 2011;33(2):32–9.

78. van Staa AL, Jedeloo S, van Meeteren J, Latour JM. Crossing the transition chasm: experiences and recommendations for improving transitional care of young adults, parents and

providers. Child Care Health Dev. 2011a;37(6):821–32. https://doi.org/10.1111/j.1365-2214 .2011.01261.x.

79. Young NL, Barden WS, Mills WA, Burke TA, Law M, Boydell K. Transition to adult-oriented health care: perspectives of youth and adults with complex physical disabilities. Phys Occup Ther Pediatr. 2009;29(4):345–61. https://doi.org/10.3109/01942630903245994.

80. Schultz RJ. Parental experiences transitioning their adolescent with epilepsy and cognitive impairments to adult health care. J Pediatr Health Care. 2013;27(5):359–66. https://doi. org/10.1016/j.pedhc.2012.03.004.

81. Berkowitz S, Lang P. Transitioning patients with complex health care needs to adult practices: theory versus reality. Pediatrics. 2020;145(6):e20193943. https://doi.org/10.1542/ peds.2019-3943.

82. Bratt EL, Burström Å, Hanseus K, Rydberg A, Berghammer M. Do not forget the parents—parents' concerns during transition to adult care for adolescents with congenital heart disease. Child Care Health Dev. 2018;44(2):278–84. https://doi.org/10.1111/cch.12529.

83. Coyne I, Malone H, Chubb E, While AE. Transition from paediatric to adult healthcare for young people with cystic fibrosis: parents' information needs. J Child Health Care. 2018;22(4):646–57. https://doi.org/10.1177/1367493518768448.

84. Coyne I, Sheehan A, Heery E, While AE. Healthcare transition for adolescents and young adults with long-term conditions: qualitative study of patients, parents and healthcare professionals' experiences. J Clin Nurs. 2019;28(21–22):4062–76. https://doi.org/10.1111/ jocn.15006.

85. Franklin MS, Beyer LN, Brotkin SM, Maslow GR, Pollock MD, Docherty SL. Health care transition for adolescent and young adults with intellectual disability: views from the parents. J Pediatr Nurs. 2019;47:148–58. https://doi.org/10.1016/j.pedn.2019.05.008.

86. Holtz BE, Mitchell KM, Holmstrom AJ, Cotten SR, Hershey DD, Dunneback JK, Jimenez Vega J, Wood MA. Teen and parental perspectives regarding transition of care in type 1 diabetes. Children Youth Serv Rev. 2020;110:104800. https://doi.org/10.1016/j. childyouth.2020.104800.

87. Thomsen EL, Khoury LR, Møller T, Boisen KA. Parents to chronically ill adolescents have ambivalent views on confidential youth consultations – a mixed methods study. Int J Adolesc Med Health. 2019; https://doi.org/10.1515/ijamh-2018-0226.

88. Wright J, Elwell L, McDonagh JE, Kelly DA, Wray J. Parents in transition: experiences of parents of young people with a liver transplant transferring to adult services. Pediatr Transplant. 2017;21(1):e12760. https://doi.org/10.1111/petr.12760.

89. Ambresin AE, Bennett K, Patton GC, Sanci LA, Sawyer SM. Assessment of youth-friendly health care: a systematic review of indicators drawn from young people's perspectives. J Adolesc Health. 2013;52(6):670–81. https://doi.org/10.1016/j.jadohealth.2012.12.014.

90. Department of Health. You're welcome: quality criteria for young people friendly services. London: Department of Health; 2011.

91. Hargreaves DS, McDonagh JE, Viner RM. Validation of you're welcome quality criteria for adolescent health services using data from national inpatient surveys in England. J Adolesc Health. 2013;52(1):50–57.e1. https://doi.org/10.1016/j.jadohealth.2012.04.005.

92. Sawyer SM, Ambresin AE, Bennett KE, Patton GC. A measurement framework for quality health care for adolescents in hospital. J Adolesc Health. 2014;55(4):484–90. https://doi. org/10.1016/j.jadohealth.2014.01.023.

93. Farre A, Wood V, McDonagh JE, Parr JR, Reape D, Rapley T, On Behalf of the Transition Collaborative Group. Health professionals' and managers' definitions of developmentally appropriate healthcare for young people: conceptual dimensions and embedded controversies. Arch Dis Child. 2016;101(7):628–33. https://doi.org/10.1136/archdischild-2015-309473.

94. Smith J, Kendal S. Parents' and health professionals' views of collaboration in the management of childhood long-term conditions. J Pediatr Nurs. 2018;43:36–44. https://doi. org/10.1016/j.pedn.2018.08.01.

95. McDonagh JE, Southwood TR, Shaw KL. The impact of a coordinated transitional care programme on adolescents with juvenile idiopathic arthritis. Rheumatology. 2007;46(1):161–8. https://doi.org/10.1093/rheumatology/kel198.
96. Shaw KL, Watanabe A, Rankin E, McDonagh JE. Walking the talk. Implementation of transitional care guidance in a UK paediatric and a neighbouring adult facility: implementation of UK transitional care guidance. Child Care Health Dev. 2014;40(5):663–70. https://doi.org/10.1111/cch.12110.
97. Zhang LF, Ho JS, Kennedy SE. A systematic review of the psychometric properties of transition readiness assessment tools in adolescents with chronic disease. BMC Pediatr. 2014;14(1):4. https://doi.org/10.1186/1471-2431-14-4.
98. Straus EJ. Challenges in measuring healthcare transition readiness: taking stock and looking forward. J Pediatr Nurs. 2019;46:109–17. https://doi.org/10.1016/j.pedn.2019.03.016.
99. Moynihan M, Saewyc E, Whitehouse S, Paone M, McPherson G. Assessing readiness for transition from paediatric to adult health care: revision and psychometric evaluation of the Am I ON TRAC for Adult Care questionnaire. J Adv Nurs. 2015;71(6):1324–35. https://doi.org/10.1111/jan.12617.
100. Nagra A, McGinnity PM, Davis N, Salmon AP. Implementing transition: ready steady go. Archiv Dis Childhood Educ Pract. 2015;100(6):313–20. https://doi.org/10.1136/archdischild-2014-307423.
101. Trapeze: a supported leap into adult health. The Sydney Children's Hospitals Network. http://www.trapeze.org.au/.
102. Fredericks EM, Dore-Stites D, Well A, Magee JC, Freed GL, Shieck V, Lopez MJ. Assessment of transition readiness skills and adherence in pediatric liver transplant recipients. Pediatr Transplant. 2010;14(8):944–53. https://doi.org/10.1111/j.1399-3046.2010.01349.x.
103. Kaugars AS, Kichler JC, Alemzadeh R. Assessing readiness to change the balance of responsibility for managing type 1 diabetes mellitus: adolescent, mother, and father perspectives. Pediatr Diabetes. 2011;12(6):547–55. https://doi.org/10.1111/j.1399-5448.2010.00737.x.
104. Gilleland J, Amaral S, Mee L, Blount R. Getting ready to leave: transition readiness in adolescent kidney transplant recipients. J Pediatr Psychol. 2012;37(1):85–96. https://doi.org/10.1093/jpepsy/jsr049.
105. McDonagh JE, Farre A. Transitional care in rheumatology: a review of the literature from the past 5 years. Curr Rheumatol Rep. 2019;21(10):57. https://doi.org/10.1007/s11926-019-0855-4.
106. Kuo D, Houtrow A, Arango P, Kuhlthau K, Simmons J, Neff J. Family centered care: current applications and future directions in pediatric health care. J Matern Child Health. 2012;16(2):297–305. https://doi.org/10.1007/s10995-011-0751-7.
107. Paul M, O'Hara L, Tah P, Street C, Maras A, Purper-Ouakil D, Santosh P, Signorini G, Singh SP, Tuomainen H, McNicholas F, For the MILESTONE Consortium. A systematic review of the literature on ethical aspects of transitional care between child- and adult-orientated health services. BMC Med Ethics. 2018;19(1):73. https://doi.org/10.1186/s12910-018-0276-3.
108. Hullmann SE, Wolfe-Christensen C, Ryan JL, Fedele DA, Rambo PL, Chaney JM, Mullins LL. Parental overprotection, perceived child vulnerability, and parenting stress: a cross-illness comparison. J Clin Psychol Med Settings. 2010;17(4):357–65. https://doi.org/10.1007/s10880-010-9213-4.
109. Carpentier MY, Mullins LL, Chaney JM, Wagner JL. The relationship of illness uncertainty and attributional style to long-term psychological distress in parents of children with Type 1 Diabetes Mellitus. Child Health Care. 2006;35(2):141–54. https://doi.org/10.1207/s15326888chc3502_3.
110. Chaney JM, Gamwell KL, Baraldi AN, Ramsey RR, Cushing CC, Mullins AJ, Gillaspy SR, Jarvis JN, Mullins LL. Parent perceptions of illness uncertainty and children depressive symptoms in juvenile rheumatic diseases: examining caregiver demand and parent distress as mediators. J Pediatr Psychol. 2016;41(9):941–51. https://doi.org/10.1093/jpepsy/jsw004.

111. Hinton D, Kirk S. Living with uncertainty and hope: a qualitative study exploring parent's experiences of living with childhood multiple sclerosis. Chronic Illn. 2017;13(2):88–99. https://doi.org/10.1177/1742395316664959.

112. Han PKJ, Klein WMP, Arora NK. Varieties of uncertainty in healthcare: a conceptual taxonomy. Med Decis Making. 2011;31(6):828–38. https://doi.org/10.1177/0272989x11393976.

113. Maslow GR, Chung RJ. Systematic review of positive youth development programs for adolescents with chronic illness. Pediatrics. 2013;131:e1605–18. https://doi.org/10.1542/peds.2012-1615.

114. Hilberink SR, Grootoonk A, Ketelaar M, Vos I, Cornet L, Roebroeck ME. Focus on autonomy: using 'Skills for Growing Up' in pediatric rehabilitation care. J Pediatr Rehabil Med. 2020;13(2):151–67. https://doi.org/10.3233/PRM-190618.

115. Hilberink SR, van Ool M, van der Stege HA, van Vliet MC, van Heijningen-Tousain HJM, de Louw AJ, van Staa AL. Skills for growing up-epilepsy: an exploratory mixed methods study into a communication tool to promote autonomy and empowerment of youth with epilepsy. Epilepsy Behav. 2018;86:116–23. https://doi.org/10.1016/j.yebeh.2018.05.040.

116. Sattoe JNT, Hilberink SR, Peeters MAC, van Staa AL. 'Skills for Growing Up': supporting autonomy in young people with kidney disease. J Ren Care. 2014;40(2):131–9. https://doi.org/10.1002/jorc.12046.

117. van Staa AL, van der Stege HA, Jedeloo S, Moll HA, Hilberink SR. Readiness to transfer to adult care of adolescents with chronic conditions: exploration of associated factors. J Adolesc Health. 2011b;48(3):295–302. https://doi.org/10.1016/j.jadohealth.2010.07.009.

118. Law E, Fisher E, Eccleston C, Palermo TM. Psychological interventions for parents of children and adolescents with chronic illness. Cochrane Database Syst Rev. 2019;3(3):CD009660. https://doi.org/10.1002/14651858.CD009660.pub4.

119. Bradshaw S, Bem D, Shaw K, Taylor B, Chiswell C, Salama M, Bassett E, Kaur G, Cummins C. Improving health, wellbeing and parenting skills in parents of children with special health care needs and medical complexity – a scoping review. BMC Pediatr. 2019;19(1):301. https://doi.org/10.1186/s12887-019-1648-7.

120. Johnson G, Kent G, Leather J. Strengthening the parent-child relationship: a review of family interventions and their use in medical settings. Child Care Health Dev. 2005;31(1):25–32. https://doi.org/10.1111/j.1365-2214.2005.00446.x.

121. Ainbinder JG, Blanchard LW, Singer GHS, Sullivan ME, Powers LK, Marquis JG, Santelli B. A qualitative study of parent to parent support for parents of children with special needs. J Pediatr Psychol. 1998;23(2):99–109. https://doi.org/10.1093/jpepsy/23.2.99.

122. Ireys HT, Chernoff R, Stein REK, DeVet KA, Silver EJ. Outcomes of community-based family-to-family support: lessons learned from a decade of randomized trials. Child Serv. 2001;4(4):203–16. https://doi.org/10.1207/S15326918CS0404_04.

123. Kingsnorth S, Gall C, Beayni S, Rigby P. Parents as transition experts? Qualitative findings from a pilot parent-led peer support group. Child Care Health Dev. 2011;37(6):833–40. https://doi.org/10.1111/j.1365-2214.2011.01294.x.

124. Law M, King S, Stewart D, King G. The perceived effects of parent-led support groups for parents of children with disabilities. Phys Occup Ther Pediatr. 2001;21(2–3):29–48. https://doi.org/10.1067/mpd.2003.138.

125. Martin S, Struemph KL, Poblete A, Toledo-Tamula MA, Lockridge R, Roderick MC, Wolters P. An Internet support group for parents of children with neurofibromatosis type 1: a qualitative analysis. J Community Genet. 2018;9(3):327–34. https://doi.org/10.1007/s12687-018-0360-x.

126. Shilling V, Morris C, Thompson-Coon J, Ukoumunne O, Rogers M, Logan S. Peer support for parents of children with chronic disabling conditions: a systematic review of quantitative and qualitative studies. Dev Med Child Neurol. 2013;55(7):602–9. https://doi.org/10.1111/dmcn.12091.

127. Towns SJ, Bell SC. Transition of adolescents with cystic fibrosis from paediatric to adult care. Clin Respir J. 2011;5(2):64–75. https://doi.org/10.1111/j.1752-699X.2010.00226.x.

128. Akré C, Polvinen J, Ullrich NJ, Rich M. Children's at home: pilot study assessing dedicated social media for parents of adolescents with neurofibromatosis type 1. J Genet Couns. 2018;27(2):505–17. https://doi.org/10.1007/s10897-018-0213-0.

129. Shilling V, Bailey S, Logan S, Morris C. Peer support for parents of disabled children. Part 1: perceived outcomes of a one-to-one service, a qualitative study. Child Care Health Dev. 2015a;41(4):524–36. https://doi.org/10.1111/cch.12223.

130. Shilling V, Bailey S, Logan S, Morris C. Peer support for parents of disabled children. Part 2: how organizational and process factors influenced shared experience in a one-to-one service, a qualitative study. Child Care Health Dev. 2015b;41(4):537–46. https://doi.org/10.1111/cch.12222.

131. Bray L, Carter B, Sanders C, Blake L, Keegan K. Parent-to-parent peer support for parents of children with a disability: a mixed method study. Patient Educ Couns. 2017;100(8):1537–43. https://doi.org/10.1016/j.pec.2017.03.004.

132. Donegan A, Boyle B, Crandall W, Dotson JL, Lemont C, Moon T, Kim SC. Connecting families: a pediatric IBD center's development and implementation of a volunteer parent mentor program. Inflamm Bowel Dis. 2016;22(5):1151–6. https://doi.org/10.1097/MIB.0000000000000733.

133. Early TJ, Glenmaye LF. Valuing families: social work practice with families from a strengths perspective. Soc Work. 2000;45:118–30. https://doi.org/10.1093/sw/45.2.118.

134. Buford TA. Transfer of asthma management responsibility from parents to their school-age children. J Pediatr Nurs. 2004;19(1):3–12. https://doi.org/10.1016/j.pedn.2003.09.002.

135. Giarelli E, Bernhardt BA, Mack R, Pyeritz RE. Adolescents' transition to self-management of a chronic genetic disorder. Qual Health Res. 2008;18(4):441–57. https://doi.org/10.1177/1049732308314853.

136. Hanna KM, Guthrie D. Parents' and adolescents' perceptions of helpful and nonhelpful support for adolescents' assumption of diabetes management responsibility. Issues Compr Pediatr Nurs. 2001;24(4):209–23. https://doi.org/10.1080/014608601753260317.

137. Aldiss S, Ellis J, Cass H, Pettigrew T, Rose L, Gibson F. Transition from child to adult care – 'it's not a one-off event': development of benchmarks to improve the experience. J Pediatr Nurs. 2015;30(5):638–47. https://doi.org/10.1016/j.pedn.2015.05.020.

138. INVOLVE. Co-production in action: number one. Southampton: INVOLVE; 2019. https://www.invo.org.uk/wp-content/uploads/2019/07/Copro_In_Action_2019.pdf.

139. Aquino E, Bristol TE, Crowe V, DesGeorges J, Heinrich P. Powerful partnerships: a handbook for families and providers working together to improve care [PDF]. Boston: National Initiative for Children's Healthcare Quality (NICHQ); 2012. https://www.nichq.org/resource/powerful-partnerships-handbookfamilies-and-providers-working-together-improve-care.

140. Bartholomew LK, Parcel GS, Kok G. Intervention mapping: a process for developing theory- and evidence-based health education programs. Health Educ Behav. 1998;25(5):545–63. https://doi.org/10.1177/109019819802500502.

141. Craig P, Dieppe P, Macintyre S, Michie S, Nazareth I, Petticrew M. Developing and evaluating complex interventions: the new medical research council guidance. Int J Nurs Stud. 2013;50(5):587–92. https://doi.org/10.1016/j.ijnurstu.2012.09.010.

142. Michie S, van Stralen MM, West R. The behaviour change wheel: a new method for characterising and designing behaviour change interventions. Implement Sci. 2011;6:42. https://doi.org/10.1186/1748-5908-6-42.

143. Powell BJ, Beidas RS, Lewis CC, Aarons GA, McMillen JC, Proctor EK, Mandell DS. Methods to improve the selection and tailoring of implementation strategies. J Behav Health Serv Res. 2017;44(2):177–94. https://doi.org/10.1007/s11414-015-9475-6.

Susan Kirk and Linda J. Milnes

7.1   Introduction

Children and young people with chronic conditions experience poorer psychosocial and educational outcomes than their healthy peers and report a range of emotional problems such as depression, anxiety and social isolation [1–3]. Studies consistently describe the sense of difference young people feel and the strategies they use to manage this experience [4–8]. Peer support has been proposed as a solution to reducing feelings of loneliness and difference and to promoting self-management [9]. In this chapter, we will argue that adolescence is a particularly appropriate time for peer support given the importance of peers in young peoples' lives, including those living with a chronic condition. We will start by analysing definitions of 'peer' and peer support; examining the key components of peer support and its different types. The theoretical underpinnings of peer support will be explored and a typology will be proposed that can be used to categorise programmes and interventions. We will present a logic model that explains the hypothesised relationship between peer support and improvements in health and wellbeing. Following on from this we will then examine the research evidence in relation to two key issues: firstly, whether peer support improves the health and wellbeing of young people with chronic conditions (i.e. effectiveness) and secondly, our understandings of young peoples' views on peer support (i.e. acceptability). The chapter concludes by considering the risks of peer support and the criticisms that have been directed at it before highlighting the implications for practice and research that arise from our current knowledge-base.

S. Kirk (✉)
School of Health Sciences, Faculty of Biology, Medicine and Health, University of
Manchester, Manchester, UK
e-mail: sue.kirk@manchester.ac.uk

L. J. Milnes
School of Healthcare, Faculty of Medicine and Heath, University of Leeds, Leeds, UK

© Springer Nature Switzerland AG 2021   135
J. N. T. Sattoe et al. (eds.), *Self-Management of Young People with Chronic
Conditions*, https://doi.org/10.1007/978-3-030-64293-8_7

7.2   Background

The number of children and young people living with a chronic condition has increased significantly in recent decades with estimates that approximately 12% of young people aged 10–19 years now have a chronic condition [2, 10]. Indeed, recent research in the United Kingdom (UK) suggests that 23% of young people aged 11–15 define themselves as having a chronic condition or disability [11]. At the same time there is evidence to suggest that they experience poorer psychosocial and educational outcomes when compared to their healthy peers [1, 3, 12–14]. Studies have reported that young people with chronic conditions may experience a range of emotional and behavioural problems such as anxiety, depression, anger, social isolation, loneliness and low self-esteem [2, 4, 8, 15]. Studies have also highlighted that there can be challenges in engaging young people in following treatment management plans which may lead to short- and long-term health complications [16, 17].

Research exploring young peoples' experiences of living with different chronic conditions has revealed consistent themes and illuminates potential contributory factors in relation to the evidence about negative psychosocial outcomes. The literature highlights how living with a chronic condition involves managing physical symptoms such as pain and living a life structured around treatment regimens [4, 6, 8, 18–23]. Young people describe a sense of being controlled by their condition and its associated management [20, 21]. However, overtime as they become increasingly responsible for self-management and treatment regimens this may provide them with a sense of mastery and control [5, 6].

Nevertheless, the treatment regimens associated with their health condition along with physical limitations and possible visible impairments can lead young people to experience a sense of difference [4, 6–8, 20, 24–27]. Despite this, it is also apparent that they strive to perceive and present themselves as 'normal' (i.e. non-different to their healthy peers) [4, 5, 8, 20, 24–26, 28]. Consequently, young people use different strategies to achieve a sense of normality and peer acceptance. To minimise the disruption of therapeutic regimens and to keep their illness in the background of their lives, young people may stop or adapt treatments in order to present a 'normal' social identify [5, 25]. Another strategy is reframing their sense of normality using downward social comparison in order to perceive themselves as fortunate and adjust to a sense of difference from their healthy peers [4, 6, 8, 18, 22]. However, the most commonly cited strategy for managing difference appears to be concealment. Studies describe how, where possible, young people conceal their condition and difference from others [25–27, 29, 30]. It has been proposed that peer support may have the potential to positively influence the psychosocial and health outcomes of young people with a chronic condition by reducing their feelings of loneliness and difference and increasing their motivation and knowledge for self-management [9]. Moreover, it has been argued that adolescence is a particularly appropriate developmental stage to introduce peer support due to the increasing importance of peers in young peoples' lives [31].

While peer-led education in school settings can be traced back to the nineteenth century [32], the origins of peer support in a health care context lie in the consumer-led self-help movement which developed in response to dissatisfaction with health care systems [33]. Central to the self-help movement was lay leadership, where peers with experiential knowledge extended existing social networks and complemented professional health services [33]. Subsequently health services themselves began to incorporate peers in delivering services for different populations. In relation to physical chronic conditions, the most well-known examples are peer-led structured self-management programmes such as the Chronic Disease Self-Management Program (United States of America (USA)), Arthritis Self-management Programme (Australia) and the Expert Patient's Programme (UK) [34]. While the first programmes were designed for adults these were subsequently extended to adolescents (e.g. Staying Positive in the UK) [34].

In terms of research, peer support has been examined in relation to both adults (including parents) and children and young people and in relation to a wide range of contexts such as developmental life transitions (e.g. pregnancy); loss (e.g. bereavement); addiction; health promotion, illness prevention and chronic conditions [33]. In relation to children and young people, peer support has been examined in the context of health promotion [35, 36], mental health [37–39], disability [40–43] and chronic physical health conditions [44, 45]. This chapter will focus on examining peer support for young people with chronic physical conditions such as asthma and diabetes and will not include parent peer support in this context.

7.3 Peer Relationships and Young People with Chronic Conditions

Developmentally adolescence is a time of transition where the key influencers on a young person's life move from being their parents to their peers [46, 47]. Indeed, peer relationships are believed to be more important during adolescence than at any other stage of life [48]. Peers are a site of socialisation for young people where they develop their self-identity, self-efficacy and their sense of belonging and status [48–51]. This entails responding to the influence (and pressure) of the group in order to gain and maintain acceptance and approval [48]. Consequently, peers may influence behaviour and wellbeing both positively and negatively [46, 48, 50, 52]. Increasingly though we are becoming aware that peers may be an important source of social support for young people [46, 47, 53].

Research has highlighted the importance of peer acceptance and friendships for young people with chronic conditions [4, 6, 25, 26, 47, 54]. Indeed, friends can be an important source of emotional and practical support and may influence self-management both positively and negatively [44, 46, 47, 52, 55–57]. However, there is also evidence that young people with chronic conditions can encounter bullying that is associated with their illness [3, 25, 54, 58]. Disclosure of their condition to others is a particularly challenging issue for young people to negotiate due to the uncertainty around peer responses [29, 58, 59]. In addition, school absences and difficulties participating in social activities may create barriers to developing and maintaining friendships [3, 6, 19, 23, 25, 54, 60]. Studies suggest that opportunities to meet with other young people with the same condition are valued due to the sense of normalcy created which reduces feelings of isolation and difference as well as providing an opportunity to share experiences and develop knowledge and ways of coping [4, 25, 26, 61, 62]. Consequently, it is not surprising that the potential benefits of developing peer support programmes for young people with chronic conditions have been recognised [49, 56].

7.4   What Is Peer Support?

Before examining the definitions of peer support, its components and categorisation, it is important to consider how the term 'peer' is defined. The Oxford English Dictionary [63] defines a peer as a

> *Person who equals another in natural gifts, ability, or achievements; the equal in any respect of a person or thing. A member of the same age group or social set; a contemporary*

The sharing of common characteristics such as age, gender, health condition as well as the notion of equality are consistently present in how 'peer' is defined in the peer support literature [41, 48, 64]. Dennis [33] has developed the definition of peer further to include more specific features relevant to our understanding of how 'peer' has been conceptualised in relation to peer support, in particular in relation to the nature of peer knowledge:

> *The peer is a created source of support, internal to a community, who shares salient target population similarities (e.g. age, ethnicity, health concern, or stressor) and possesses specific knowledge that is concrete, pragmatic, present-oriented, and derived from personal experience rather than formal training.*

Dennis's [33] definition of peer support within a health care context combines the particular nature of knowledge possessed by a peer and their shared characteristics along with the types of support that are exchanged:

> *The provision of emotional, appraisal, and informational assistance by a created social network member who possesses experiential knowledge of a specific behaviour or stressor and similar characteristics as the target population, to address a health-related issue of a potentially or actually stressed focal person.*

It is important to note that in the literature the term 'peer support' may be used interchangeably with terms such as 'peer education', 'peer befriending', 'peer buddying' and 'peer mentoring' or as an umbrella term encompassing all of these latter terms [36, 38, 65]. There can however be differences in emphasis. For example, peer mentoring, which is a common approach of many peer support programmes for children and young people, characterises the peer mentor as being older than the young person, as having similar life or illness experiences and as receiving formalised training to prepare them for their role [36, 45, 49, 66].

7.4.1   Peer Support: Components and Categories

Five key components of peer support are evident in the literature. Firstly, as evident in the definitions of a peer, a key component is the possession of similar character-istics such as age, ethnicity, life situation or health condition [53, 67]. Secondly, and related to the first component, the provision of peer support is based on knowledge gained through direct experience (for example, of living with a chronic condition) [53, 64, 65, 67]. Thirdly, a set of values underpin and shape the peer relationship: respect, autonomy, equality, personalisation and empowerment [64, 65, 68–70]. Fourthly, the relationship is one of reciprocity and mutuality where the giving and receiving of help and the sharing of experiences is seen as benefitting both parties [65, 68, 69]; in addition, there is a shared responsibility and mutual agreement about what is helpful [64, 70]. Finally, peer support is goal orientated; it aims to bring about a desired personal or social change [65, 69]. In relation to living with a chronic condition this could include improving health and wellbeing, enhancing self-management or adjusting to life with a chronic condition [16, 71].

Three categories or types of peer support have been identified [9, 16, 33, 67]. *Emotional Support* which involves providing encouragement, reassurance and opportunities for reflection while demonstrating caring, empathy and active listen-ing. This form of support is aimed at bolstering self-esteem and fostering feelings of acceptance, being cared for, respected, understood and valued. *Informational sup-port* which is the provision of knowledge to enable problem-solving, decision-making and action. It involves providing information, advice and suggestions about resources and possible actions related to a particular topic or issue that the individ-ual is facing. The third category of support is *appraisal* or *affirmational support* which involves providing feedback to the individual that affirms the appropriateness of their feelings, thoughts and behaviours. It involves motivating and encouraging the person to persevere with their attempts at managing the issues they face despite setbacks, helping them to tolerate frustration and develop and maintain an optimis-tic and positive outlook.

7.5   Theoretical Underpinnings of Peer Support

Explanations for the link between peer support and improvements in health and wellbeing have been informed by different social and psychological theories [33, 69]. These include the Transactional Theory of Stress and Coping [72]; Social Learning Theory [73]; and Social Support [74]. Figure 7.1 summarises how peer support has been theorised to influence health outcomes.

It has been proposed that peer support influences health outcomes via different mechanisms [33, 49, 64]. Firstly, that the peer relationship developed reduces feel-ings of isolation, loneliness, alienation, low self-esteem and loss of control and improves social integration. Secondly, that peer support involves the provision of information which positively influences health behaviours. Thirdly, that peer sup-port motivates positive self-care, help-seeking and adherence to medical regimens

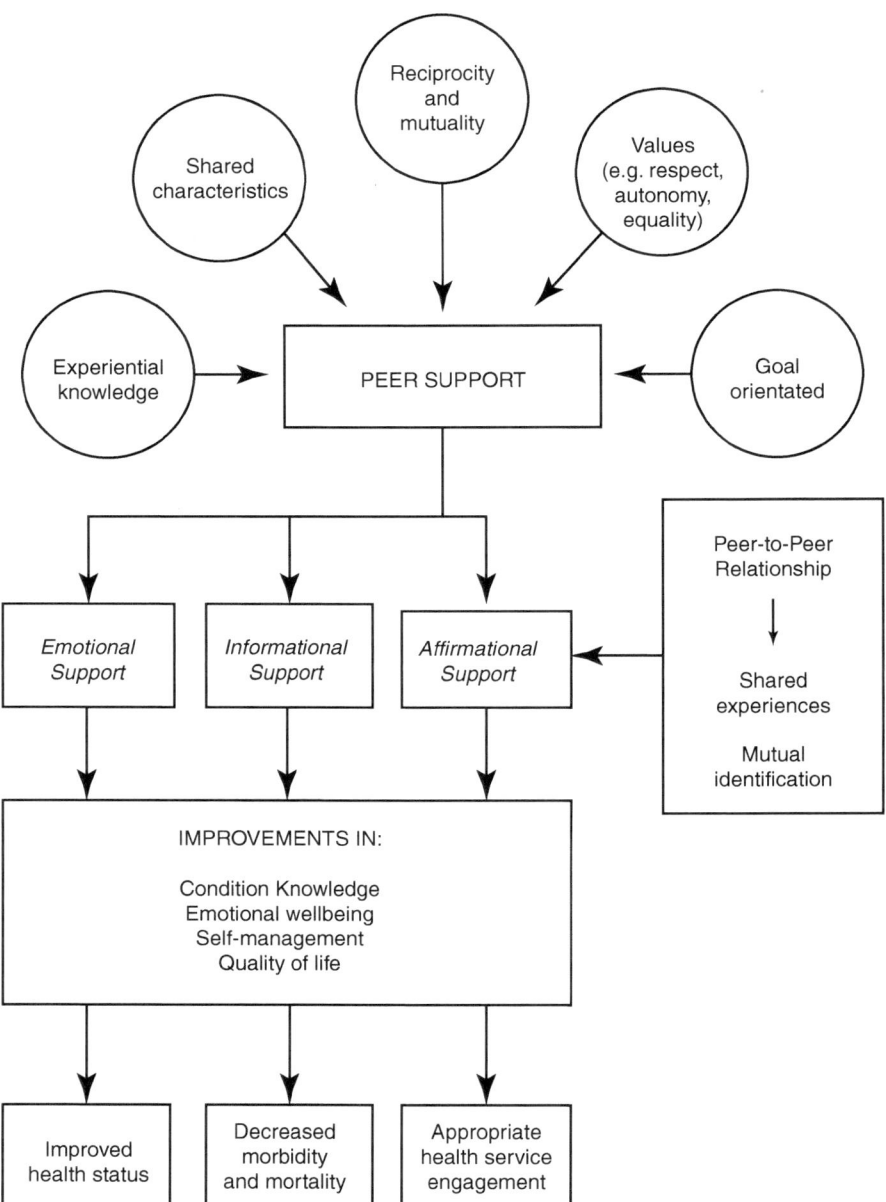

Fig. 7.1 The influence of peer support on health outcomes

and promotes a positive outlook. Therefore, peer support is seen as acting as a buffer; protecting individuals from stress and negative stimuli and influencing their responses to these stimuli [33, 65]. It is also been theorised that peer support acts as a mediator influencing health indirectly by influencing emotions, cognitions and behaviours; for example, through teaching coping strategies [33].

As noted earlier peer support is also underpinned by certain assumptions about peer-to-peer relationships and interactions and how these promote wellbeing. At the centre of peer support is a shared experience which makes it distinctive to the support provided by health care professionals. This shared experience is cited as providing access to experiential knowledge; knowledge and insights that are based on direct experience which is unavailable to professionals [49, 71]. Possessing a shared experience is viewed as being the basis for a greater understanding of the particular challenges/situation faced by an individual and as a consequence a more authentic empathy than that provided by others in an individuals' embedded social networks [33, 65, 68]. Mutual identification is also presented as being inherent in the peer-to-peer relationship with the ability to identify with one another which promotes credibility and trustworthiness [34, 64, 65, 69]. Observing peers and witnessing them share and disclose personal experiences and manage their daily lives is seen as reducing feelings of isolation, difference and stigma and promoting feelings of normalcy, belonging and hope [34, 49, 69, 71]. This in turn increases the motivation to achieve personal goals [69].

7.6   Peer Support Models and Programmes

Peer support is described as being a 'wellness model' that focuses on peoples' strengths and abilities rather than being an illness or deficit model which accentuates symptoms and problems [65, 75]. It has also been categorised as a social support model due to its emphasis on the support derived from social relationships and connections [64, 66]. There are three broad models of peer support [33, 65, 67]. Firstly, informal or naturally occurring peer support, for example, support from friends. Secondly, peer support that arises from participation in consumer or peer-led programmes. Thirdly, the employment of consumers/service users as providers of services/support within traditional services. In this chapter, we will focus on the second broad model.

There is a large variation in peer support programmes in relation to their aims; their target group; the programme's content/activities; the duration of the programme; the mode or medium of delivery; their location/setting; and the role, training and support of peer facilitators [9, 16, 38, 71]. Figure 7.2 presents a typology for peer support programmes based on the literature which can be used to characterise individual programmes or interventions [9, 16, 33, 38, 57, 67, 68].

In relation to young people living with chronic conditions, some self-management or self-care programmes include peer support components [76–79]. An example is

DIMENSTION	DESCRIPTION
Peer-to-Peer Relationship	Peer on the basis of age, condition or age and condition.
Target	Specific health condition or range of health conditions.
Setting	Home, school, hospital, clinic, camp, community organisation
Provider	Consumer/charity organisation, community or hospital-based helath care organisations
Mode of Delivery	Individual or group based
Medium of Delivery	Telephone-based, Internet-based, Face to face, combination
Peer Role	Educator, advocate, leader, counsellor, mediator, linking agent, or cultural tanslator. Training and support of peer facilitators.
Nature of the Programme	Aims of programme Content and activities Duration of programme Degree of structure: highly formalised, informal and individualised. Degree of peer support: primary programme, component of a wider programme.

Fig. 7.2 A typology for peer support programmes

a problem-solving and social skills development programme developed for young people with cystic fibrosis that combined an individualised home-based educational programme with peer group activities and discussion [80]. As we will discuss later, programmes focussing on the provision of peer support have been developed for those with a specific health condition (for example, asthma, diabetes, Juvenile Idiopathic Arthritis, HIV) as well as generic programmes designed to be appropriate for young people with various chronic conditions.

Three broad approaches to providing peer support are evident in studies that have evaluated peer support programmes for young people with chronic conditions: therapeutic camps, face-to-face programmes and online peer support. Although as we will see, within these three approaches there is substantial variability in the programmes developed and evaluated.

7.6.1   Therapeutic Camps

Therapeutic camps for young people with chronic conditions are particularly preva-lent in North America which has a long-standing history of organised residential Summer camps for children. While therapeutic camps vary in design, location and duration, they usually aim to enable young people to participate in recreational and leisure activities in a safe environment, away from their families but supervised by health care professionals and sometimes by adults with the same condition who act as role models. Most camps focus on a single condition and aim to promote inde-pendence and self-esteem; provide social support and education; and opportunities to engage in skills building [81, 82]. This may occur through informal peer interac-tions or through providing formal education sessions [81]. While some studies have evaluated peer-led self-management programmes that are provided in a camp set-ting [44, 52], most studies have evaluated the overall camp experience [56, 81, 83–88]. Although most studies have been conducted in a North American context, there are examples of camps being evaluated in Ireland [87, 88], The Netherlands [56] and the UK [86].

7.6.2   Face-to-Face Programmes

Various face-to-face peer support programmes have been developed and evaluated which differ in relation to the degree of structure imposed on the provision of peer support. Structured, group-based programmes include: the Triple A Programme which is a three-step school-based peer-led programme that aims to educate and empower young people about asthma and its management (including those with an asthma diagnosis) [89–91]; and 'Staying Positive' a generic, peer-led, programme based on the Stanford Chronic Disease Self-management programme that aims to improve young people's confidence in managing their condition and improve their psychosocial wellbeing [92]. Other structured group-based programmes have been developed and evaluated for young people with diabetes [93], asthma [17] and heart disease [94] but are led by professionals rather than peers. Not all face-to-face pro-grammes are group based; in a one-to-one, peer support programme peer leaders used planned motivational interviewing to improve young people's engagement with HIV services [95]. Another one-to-one programme was unstructured with peer mentors organising individualised activities to promote self-management and psy-chosocial wellbeing for young liver transplant recipients alongside communication via text messaging, e-mail, or social media [96]. Other less structured group-based peer support programmes are those where the programme's content is formulated by the participants themselves [71, 97, 98]. An example of this is the Chronic Illness Peer Support (ChIPS) which is a long-standing, 8-week programme for young peo-ple with any chronic condition that includes regular social events [71, 98]. The programme is jointly led by older peers and health professional facilitators and aims to improve adjustment to living with a chronic illness, develop participants' personal abilities, increase their sense of control over their health and become more active in their local community.

These face-to-face programmes differ from therapeutic camps which are traditionally residential and include a wide range of recreational and leisure activities as a means of achieving their goals. However, as noted above some formalised peer self-management programmes have been evaluated within a camp context, though it is unclear whether these programmes were designed to be integrated within this environment or whether the camps provided a convenient setting to evaluate their effectiveness.

7.6.3   Online Peer Support

In recent years, there has been recognition of the potential of the Internet to facilitate an accessible means of providing peer support for young people with chronic conditions. One area of progress is in the development and evaluation of online peer mentorship programmes. An example is the iPeer2Peer Program which is an online one-to-one peer mentoring program for adolescents with Juvenile Idiopathic Arthritis [45, 99]. Over an 8-week period young people engage in ten Skype video calls with peer mentors that aim to provide individualised informational, appraisal, and emotional support. The peer mentors act as positive role models to help reinforce self-management alongside social support. Other online programmes may be more structured, incorporating timetabled group-based peer mentorship sessions on specific topics [57, 100, 101]. These three examples, developed by the same team, are directed at young people with asthma and aim to improve social support and support seeking and to reduce social isolation. In two of the programmes there was professional oversight or co-facilitation [57, 101]. In addition, these more structured programmes may include a chat room or discussion board for young people to 'meet socially' between group meetings [57, 100].

Some studies have created online communities to provide peer support and have explored participants' experiences of receiving peer support via this medium and the nature of the support provided and received [102, 103]. Other studies have observed peer support within existing online communities [104, 105]. In addition, online peer support may be a component of online self-management programmes [106]. In this example a smart phone mobile health application (mHealth app) developed to support the self-management of young people with diabetes included a chat room for peer interaction and support.

7.7   Does Peer Support Improve Health and Wellbeing?

As discussed earlier in the chapter the underlying assumption of peer support programmes is that they improve participants' health and wellbeing. But what is the evidence for this in relation to young people with chronic conditions? In this section we will consider this question based on selected literature reviews and primary research studies that have investigated the effectiveness of peer support programmes. As we will see the research findings are inconsistent and the variation in programmes creates difficulties in making comparisons and synthesising findings from evaluations [9, 107]. Studies investigating the effectiveness of programmes have used different designs: experimental (randomised controlled trials (RCT)), quasi-experimental (e.g. pretest-posttest) and mixed method designs. However, this body of research has been criticised for the lack of RCTs and an over-reliance on quasi-experimental studies [9, 82, 107].

While some studies have evaluated peer support programmes directed at young people with a range of different chronic conditions (e.g. [71, 81]), many have focussed on programmes developed for a single condition such as asthma or diabetes. Indeed, peer support interventions for asthma appear to be the most frequently studied. As we have already seen there is substantial variation in the programmes apart from the condition focus. Some are pre-existing, established programmes (e.g. [56, 81]), but most are programmes developed by the researchers themselves (e.g. [44, 91]) and it is notable that only a minority of researchers report involving young people in their design and development (e.g. [57, 100]). As discussed earlier three different models of peer support can be discerned: therapeutic camps (e.g. [52, 81]); face-to-face programmes (e.g. [89, 91]) and online programmes (e.g. [45, 57]). While some programmes are peer-led, others are professionally led with the peer support element relating to the opportunity provided for interaction amongst participants (e.g. [17, 93, 94]). Programmes can also be differentiated on the basis of whether they are group (e.g. [71, 89]) or individually based (e.g. [95, 96]); structured (e.g. [17, 52, 89]) or individualised to the needs of the individual or group (e.g. [45, 96, 100]). In addition, some peer support programmes are targeted at particular ethnic groups (e.g. [17, 52]).

7.7.1 Condition-Related Knowledge

Many peer support interventions have an educational element that provides informational support with the goal of improving self-management. Studies have found young peoples' condition-related knowledge increased significantly following participation in the peer support programme [52, 89, 90, 94]. However, these differences may be clinically rather that statistically different [89] and the control groups' activities may have similarly increased participants knowledge [52, 90]. Interestingly studies have also reported significant improvements in peer leader's knowledge [108]. Systematic reviews have concluded that peer support may improve condition-related knowledge [9, 82].

7.7.2 Psychosocial Wellbeing

Peer support interventions have been associated with improvements in psychosocial wellbeing outcomes such as positive attitudes towards illness [44]; emotional wellbeing in males [91]; and decreased loneliness [57]. However, other studies report no changes in outcomes such as distress, self-esteem, loneliness and social isolation [71, 100]. Systematic reviews of therapeutic camps come to different conclusions about their potential to improve psychosocial wellbeing. One review concluded that there is evidence to suggest they improve self-esteem, self-perception, coping and reduce anxiety and distress [82], while another concludes that there is inconsistent evidence for camps having any psychosocial, cognitive, or social effects [107].

There are also inconsistent findings reported in relation to self-efficacy, with some studies reporting improvements in this outcome [56, 57, 87, 89] and others reporting no significant improvements [45, 71]. A systematic review concluded that there is evidence to suggest that peer support programmes improves self-efficacy [82]. In relation to other psychosocial wellbeing outcomes, studies report that peer support may improve: social connectedness [94]; the quality of young peoples' interactions with their parents [81]; and perceptions of support from family and friends [57]. However, another study reported no statistically significant differences in young peoples' perceptions of social support from family or friends [100]. Systematic reviews conclude that peer support interventions may improve psychosocial outcomes such as social engagement, social support and social functioning [9, 82].

7.7.3   Managing Treatment Regimens

In one study participants reported improvements in their perceived ability to manage their chronic condition following participation in a peer support programme [45]. In another study the peer mentors themselves reported clinically significant improvements in adherence although not in self-management [96]. Conversely another study found that there were no statistically significant differences in adherence between the intervention and control groups (indeed it declined in both groups) [17]. These conflicting findings are reflected in the systematic reviews, with some concluding that peer support programmes may improve adherence and self-management [9, 82], and others that the benefits for adherence remain unproven [16].

7.7.4   Quality of Life

Studies suggest that peer support interventions may improve young peoples' health-related quality of life [44, 81, 87, 89, 91, 94]. These improvements may also extend to peer leaders, as Rhee et al. [108] report significant improvements in peer leaders' quality of life. In another study participating as a peer leader had a positive effect on the independence domain of a health-related quality of life (HRQoL) measure [56]. However, other studies have found no improvements in HRQoL for participants in peer support programmes [45, 90, 93] or for peer leaders [96]. Systematic reviews conclude that there is some evidence of improvements in HRQoL in relation to therapeutic camps for young people with asthma, although these tend to be small and may be time-limited [16, 34]. A review of generic peer support interventions

concluded that there is evidence that peer support programmes improve participants' health-related quality of life [9].

7.7.5 Health Status

Health status has been measured in different ways according to the particular condition and improvements in this outcome have been reported by some researchers. In
one study diabetes control improved although only for female participants [93]. In
another study both the control and intervention group reported improvements in
lung function [91]. Some studies have found that peer leader health status may also
improve [96, 108]. However other studies have found no improvements in health
status in relation to lung function [44], pain [45] and asthma attacks [91]. Similarly,
systematic reviews conclude that there is little evidence for improvements in health
status [9, 16, 34, 107].

7.7.6 Health Service Use

The impact of peer support on health service use appears to have been under-
researched. One study reported significant differences between the intervention and
control groups in relation to health service use, with the peer-led group making
fewer acute primary care visits [109]. Taking account of this, and the reduced costs
of providing a peer-led programme, they estimated net cost savings of $51.80 over
3 months. Another study which aimed to improve engagement with services, found
that peer-led support improved the retention of young people with HIV/AIDs [95].

Returning to our question, does peer support improve health and wellbeing for
young people? The 'safest' answer currently appears to be that 'we don't know'. As
we can see there are conflicting findings and conclusions from both primary research
and systematic reviews which may not be surprising given the diversity of peer support models evaluated. Furthermore, concerns about the robustness of the quantitative research evidence have been frequently highlighted with various methodological
limitations identified [9, 16, 34, 82, 107, 110, 111]. Indeed, it may be, given the
complexity of peer support, that improvements in health and wellbeing cannot be
conclusively evaluated by experimental designs and 'gold standard' RCTs. As well
as evaluating effectiveness, researchers have also examined the important issue of
acceptability — what are young peoples' views of peer support?

7.8   Acceptability: Young Peoples' Views of Peer Support

In this section we will examine young peoples' views of peer support based on
selected literature reviews and primary research studies that have investigated this
area. In contrast to the quantitative evidence on the effectiveness of peer support
programmes, we will see that the research findings on acceptability are largely

consistent despite the variation in approaches to peer support. While studies exploring participants' perspectives have largely used qualitative research designs; either as the sole approach (e.g. [83, 84, 97]) or as a component of an experimental or mixed method study (e.g. [45, 52, 56, 71]); survey methods have also been used to obtain young peoples' views (e.g. [86, 88]).

Young peoples' perspectives have been obtained on therapeutic camps (e.g. [56, 83, 85, 86]), face-to-face programmes/groups (e.g. [71, 97]) and online programmes/groups (e.g. [101, 103, 104]). In common with studies investigating effectiveness, the body of research about acceptability has examined peer support programmes that vary in relation to whether they are: focussed on young people with a single chronic condition or are generic; are peer or professionally led; are researcher developed or established programmes; or are group or individually based. A small number of studies have also explored the experiences of peer mentors/leaders about their involvement in programmes [56, 99, 101, 108].

7.8.1 Peer Support Exchanges

Studies observing and analysing the nature of peer support interactions describe how they illustrate the provision of informational, emotional and appraisal support [49, 103, 104]. Peers share experiences and offer one another information and advice about managing illness, treatments, emotions, relationships and services [49, 103, 104]. Interactions demonstrate the development of supportive and trusting relationships and the conveyance of empathy, the building of self-esteem and participants open expression of emotions [103, 104]. It is notable that discussions extend beyond illness experiences to issues relating to being an adolescent [49]. Observations of peer interactions reveal that peer mentors have the capacity to provide mentorship to young people with chronic conditions [49].

7.8.2 Feeling Socially Connected and 'Normal'

Studies highlight how young people with chronic conditions value the opportunity to meet (either virtually or physically) with peers who share the same concerns and challenges and how this reduces their sense of isolation and difference [9, 45, 52, 56, 57, 71, 83, 84, 97, 100, 106]. In one study young people noted that it was valuable having contact with older peers who had already transitioned through the experience of living with a chronic condition during adolescence [45]. Being connected to peers is seen as enabling young people to share their feelings with individuals who understand their situation and to develop friendship networks [45, 57, 71, 84, 86, 101, 106]. In one study mentors described that they perceived that by acting as positive role models and presenting the vision of a hopeful future, increased their mentee's confidence and motivation to manage the challenges they faced [99]. Conversely one study highlighted how young people may experience the death of a peer group member which may lead to feelings of distress and concerns about their own future mortality [97].

Developing social connections with peers enables young people with chronic conditions to feel accepted and 'normal' [9, 57, 83–85, 100, 106]. Studies suggest that the development of feelings of social connection and non-difference leads young people to feel more confident in social situations [56, 57, 86, 92, 100]. For some young people maintaining relationships beyond the programme is important [57, 83, 86]. Furthermore, young people value having the opportunity to engage in enjoyable activities with others and 'have fun' [9, 52, 84–86, 92]. Although participants may find physical activities challenging [9]. Some studies have highlighted the reciprocal nature of peer support with participants describing their sense of personal satisfaction from helping others through the provision of informational and emotional support [97, 103].

One study that explored the experiences of peer mentors discovered that the process of developing a relationship between peer mentors and mentees evolved over time and was influenced by the degree of shared characteristics; the more similar the pairing were in relation to demographic characteristics then the quicker and deeper the relationship formation [99].

7.8.3 Developing Knowledge and Skills

Studies suggest that young people feel that peer support programmes develop their condition-related knowledge, coping strategies and communication skills. This occurs through the opportunity to share personal experiences and lay expertise as well as through the provision of more formalised education [9, 45, 52, 56, 57, 83, 84, 88, 92, 97, 101, 103, 106]. One study of a peer-led programme described how peer leaders were highly rated for the knowledge they possessed and for informational support they provided [108]. Mentors themselves perceive that they are viewed by young people as credible sources of support due to their personal experience of living with a chronic condition and being seen as positive role models [99, 108]. An improved understanding of their condition may lead young people to feeling more confident about managing their condition and more prepared to express their needs and seek support [56, 57, 86, 92, 100].

7.8.4 Experiences of Being a Peer Leader/Mentor

Studies exploring the experience of being a peer mentor have discovered that mentors describe it as being a rewarding experience due to the growth they witness in mentees and that this in turn improves their own personal wellbeing [99, 101, 108]. In addition, they perceive that adopting this role has increased their self-confidence and has led to personal growth [56, 99]. Indeed, the training mentors received may be regarded as a form of peer support in itself; as they report acquiring new knowledge and skills and receiving emotional support from within the peer mentor group which resulted in the development of new friendships [99]. Difficult aspects of being a peer mentor have been identified relating to logistical issues such as organising regular contact with mentees [99, 108].

7.9   The Risks and Challenges of Peer Support

Mellanby et al. [32] have highlighted how peer support models have been 'embraced with uncritical enthusiasm' with their potential problems being overlooked. Indeed, while peer support programmes have the potential to be beneficial, they may also pose risks and challenges [98]. Hearing about the problems that others are experiencing, encountering negative information about a condition, witnessing the deterioration of others can all lead to stress and distress for participants and peer workers [33, 65, 66, 98]. It has been suggested that self-efficacy and self-esteem can be reduced due to perceived criticisms from peers and negative self-appraisal resulting from social comparison if others are seen to be making greater progress [33, 98]. Furthermore, peer support may reinforce poor self-management practices and risk-taking [34]. Young people may also overidentify with and become overly emotionally attached to the peer support group and thus fail to develop other social networks and interests [33, 98]. Indeed, it has been suggested that groups may reinforce stigma through segregation as they create a 'subculture' in which participants identify themselves as being different and separate from wider society [34, 56, 90, 98, 112].

Relationships between peers may not always be positive with personality clashes and conflicts occurring [33, 66]. In peer mentorship models it has been highlighted that there may be difficulties in establishing an interpersonal connection between mentees and mentors [33, 66]. In addition, there may be boundary issues in the relationships between mentees and mentors with confusion over whether the relationship is professional or one of friendship. While peer support aims to be based on an egalitarian relationship rather than the traditional power structure of professional relationships, it has been noted that in reality the relationship is usually asymmetrical as the peer mentor possesses a level of experience unavailable to the mentee and reciprocity is minimised as the goal focusses on the growth and development of the mentee [40, 43, 65]. Moreover, this asymmetry is increased if peer workers are formally employed [65]. Indeed, concerns have been raised about the potential for the training and payment of peer workers to lead to their professionalisation and to a diversion of their accountability from the peer group to the health care system with a consequent loss of credibility and mutual identification i.e. their 'peerness' [33]. Furthermore, the risks of peer support workers being socialised into the accepted practices of the service system or following professional role models to gain respect, have been highlighted [65]. Conversely, the potential for the exploitation of peer workers has also been raised if they are used as unpaid replacements for professional services [33].

Finally, it has been questioned whether the underpinning philosophy of peer support is empowerment or compliance. Stewart et al. [57] have commented that peer support programmes often emphasise treatment compliance and clinical control rather than more psychosocial issues such as social isolation. This may be a result of the difficulty in measuring psychosocial outcomes or it could reflect the absence of a biopsychosocial underpinning philosophy and the lack of involvement of young people in coproducing interventions.

7.10   Implications and Key Recommendations for Practice and Research

This chapter has highlighted the key theoretical and research-related issues surrounding peer support for young people with chronic conditions. Despite insubstantial evidence regarding the most effective type of peer support, it remains valued as a central component and indicator of good quality self-management support in England and internationally [113–115]. In addition, existing parallels between the psychological and social skills developed during adolescence through peer relationships and the key skills required for self-management, supports the need for further research.

7.10.1 Implications for Practice

In health care practice peer support initiatives for young people with chronic conditions need to be receptive and relevant to a population with individual differences in physical, psychological and social development; culture; ethnicity; health condition; family/carer dynamics; health experiences and access to care. Due to the multiplicity of these characteristics individualised, person-centred approaches to peer support may be important components of peer support models. A flexible, integrated peer support model where young people can select from a 'menu' of different types of support, for example; individual or group-based support, online or face-to-face provision, could offer a more individualised approach. The alternative would be structured, standardised programmes that, while potentially offering a more cost-effective and efficient way of implementing peer support, lack individualisation [116]. Although there is less available evidence for young people with chronic conditions, a review of over 1000 studies identified that online discussion forums and face-to-face groups run by trained peers were the most useful types of peer support for improving emotional and physical well-being [116]. Therefore, when considering practice-based initiatives, as exemplified in personalised recovery programmes in mental health care in the UK [117], it might be helpful to focus on individualised peer support delivered either online or face-to-face.

Online formal or informal peer support can widen access for young people who live in remote areas, have rare health conditions, have limited services locally and/ or who prefer to communicate online rather than face-to-face [49, 57, 66, 101]. Informal online forms of support enable discussion topics to be raised by young people themselves rather than be pre-determined and offer immediate and responsive support for young people's 'live' problems and anxieties [104]. Moreover, despite their variability, there is some evidence for their effectiveness and acceptability [101]. One-to-one peer support from trained peer mentors appears to be a type of peer support that promotes individualisation but is dependent on the development of a positive therapeutic relationship between mentor and mentee [36, 45]. Peer mentorship has also been found to have benefits for the mentors themselves who can experience positive changes [34, 118]. However, the importance of these programmes being well resourced and providing training and ongoing support and supervision for mentors as well as being flexible for mentees means that this type of approach could be difficult to sustain in practice [36]. In addition, strategies need to be in place to manage the potential risks associated with peer support approaches described earlier in the chapter, such as challenging interpersonal relationships, emotional impact on peer mentors, and reinforcement of poor self-management practices.

Potential barriers for implementing and sustaining peer support in practice settings relate to the uncertainty of its cost-effectiveness alongside strategic and resource challenges. However, it has been suggested that peer support may be a cost-effective alternative to professionally led programmes [34], with some evidence being reported of reduced hospital use and improved health outcomes [16]. However, health-related cost-effectiveness has not yet been established, particularly over the long-term [16]. In addition, it is difficult to assess whether some peer support models can be sustained beyond the context of a research study and are feasible to implement in real-life settings [32]. Until further evidence is available and peer support more established or embedded in routine healthcare practice young people should be guided by health professionals to safe places for support, such as discussion boards on disease specific charity websites.

7.10.2 Implications for Research

Further research is needed to assess the outcomes of peer support interventions coproduced with young people and to assess how different contexts and characteristics of interventions and populations impact on the outcomes of peer support. Few studies include young people in the design and development of peer support interventions [101]. This is perhaps not surprising given a recent review found that few interventions developed to improve young peoples' health and wellbeing (including supportive interventions for chronic conditions) involved young people in codesign [119]. If peer support interventions are to be acceptable and appropriate, then it is important that young people are involved as equal partners in their coproduction. In addition, intervention development needs to be underpinned by appropriate theory. It has been suggested that the use of Positive Youth Developmental theory (a strengths-based approach) could enhance the appropriateness of peer support interventions and improve self-management, educational outcomes, interpersonal relationships and overall wellbeing [12] (Also see Chap. 2).

Further research needs to examine the influence of different characteristics in this population on the impact of peer support. The need to understand what type or variant of intervention works for different subgroups (e.g. age, ethnicity, language, gender, peer leader characteristics, condition) is commonly recommended in the literature [34, 45, 49, 110]. While there have been some suggestions in the literature that gender and family income may influence the outcomes of peer support [49, 91, 93], such correlations have not been consistently reported. Overall, an assessment of the relationship between context, causal mechanisms and outcomes in evaluations of peer support interventions is recommended [34].

The nature of peer support interventions means that they are complex both in terms of their multiple interacting components and the real-life context in which they are delivered [120]. Peer support interventions for young people include a number of different interactional components such as the mode of delivery; range of behaviours required for usage/delivery; numerous health and clinical outcomes; variability in the target population and the flexibility required for interventions to be responsive and individualised. Consequently, it is important to consider alternative research designs to randomised controlled trials for evaluation, such as mixed methods, process evaluations or realist evaluations using young person-centred approaches in order to increase our understanding of peer support interventions and their impact on young people both in the short and long term [34, 82, 107].

7.11   Conclusions

Peer support is characterised by a sharing of personal characteristics and the provision of goal-orientated support that is centred on experiential knowledge and relationships based on values such as mutuality, reciprocity, empowerment and respect. It is categorised as a strengths-based, social support model [65, 66]. While we have identified three broad peer support models for young people with chronic conditions, there are many different approaches and components to peer support as exemplified by the typology presented in the chapter (Fig. 7.2). Peer support programmes are viewed as a way of improving the health and wellbeing of young people with chronic conditions and the theory behind their mode of action is summarised (Fig. 7.1). However, the body of research investigating this relationship has reported conflicting results and has methodological limitations. Moreover, the diversity of programmes presents difficulties in making any comparisons between programmes [33, 38]. Qualitative research reports more consistent findings, suggesting that programmes are valued by young people with chronic conditions and perceived to be beneficial to health and wellbeing. Nevertheless, peer support may pose risks to young people which need to be taken into account in programme delivery. The chapter has highlighted important issues that need to be considered in developing peer support programmes: young people need to be involved in their coproduction, it is important that they are underpinned by theory and an empowerment philosophy, and that they are feasible to deliver in real-life settings. In terms of research, their level of complexity and individualisation may mean that RCTs are not viable evaluation designs and that alternative designs may be more appropriate.

References

1. Champaloux SW, Young DR. Childhood chronic health conditions and educational attainment: a social ecological approach. J Adolesc Health. 2015;56(1):98–105. https://doi.org/10.1016/j.jadohealth.2014.07.016.
2. Leeman J, Crandell JL, Lee A, Bai J, Sandelowski M, Knafl K. Family functioning and the well-being of children with chronic conditions: a meta-analysis. Res Nurs Health. 2016;39(4):229–43. https://doi.org/10.1002/nur.21725.
3. Lum CE, Wakefield B, Donnan MA, Burns JE, Fardell A, Marshall GM. Understanding the school experiences of children and adolescents with serious chronic illness: a systematic meta-review. Child Care Health Dev. 2017;43(5):645–62. https://doi.org/10.1111/cch.12475.
4. Cartwright T, Fraser E, Edmunds S, Wilkinson N, Jacobs K. Journeys of adjustment: the experiences of adolescents living with juvenile idiopathic arthritis. Child Care Health Dev. 2014;41(5):734–43. https://doi.org/10.1111/cch.12206.
5. Curtis-Tyler K. Levers and barriers to patient-centred care with children: findings from a synthesis of studies of the experiences of children living with type 1 diabetes or asthma. Child Care Health Dev. 2010;37(4):540–50. https://doi.org/10.1111/j.1365-2214.2010.01180.x.
6. Jamieson N, Fitzgerald D, Singh-Grewal D, Hanson CS, Craig JC, Tong A. Children's experiences of cystic fibrosis: a systematic review of qualitative studies. Pediatrics. 2014;133:e1683–97. https://doi.org/10.1542/peds.2014-0009.
7. Jessup M, Parkinson C. "All at sea": the experience of living with cystic fibrosis. Qual Health Res. 2010;20(3):352–64. https://doi.org/10.1177/1049732309354277.
8. Knight A, Vickery M, Fiks AG, Barg FK. The illness experience of youth with lupus/mixed connective tissue disease: a mixed methods analysis of patient and parent perspectives. Lupus. 2016;25(9):1028–39. https://doi.org/10.1177/0961203316646460.
9. Ahola Kohut S, Stinson J, van Wyk M, Giosa L, Luca S. Systematic review of peer support interventions for adolescents with chronic illness: a narrative analysis. Int J Child Adolesc Health. 2014;7(3):183–97.
10. Department of Health. Long term conditions compendium of information. 3rd ed. London: Department of Health; 2012.
11. Association for Young Peoples' Health. Key data on young people 2019. London: Association for Young Peoples' Health; 2019.
12. Maslow GR, Chung RJ. Systematic review of positive youth development programs for adolescents with chronic illness. Pediatrics. 2013;131(5):e1605–18. https://doi.org/10.1542/peds.2012-1615.
13. Nylander C, Seidel C, Tindberg Y. The triply troubled teenager - chronic conditions associated with fewer protective factors and clustered risk behaviours. Acta Paediatr. 2014;103(2):194–200. https://doi.org/10.1111/apa.12461.
14. Pinquart M, Shen Y. Depressive symptoms in children and adolescents with chronic physical illness: an updated meta-analysis. J Pediatr Psychol. 2010;36(4):375–84. https://doi.org/10.1093/jpepsy/jsq104.
15. Brady AM, Deighton J, Stansfield S. Psychiatric outcomes associated with chronic illness in adolescence: a systematic review. J Adolesc. 2017;59:112–23. https://doi.org/10.1016/j.adolescence.2017.05.014.

16. Kew KM, Carr R, Crossingham I. Lay-led and peer support interventions for adolescents with asthma. Cochrane Database Syst Rev. 2017;4:CD012331. https://doi.org/10.1002/14651858. CD012331.pub2.
17. Mosnaim G, Li H, Martin M, Richardson D, Belice P, Avery E, Ryan N, Bender B, Powell L. The impact of peer support and mp3 messaging on adherence to inhaled corticosteroids in minority adolescents with asthma: a randomized controlled trial. J Allergy Clin Immunol Pract. 2013;1(5):485–93. https://doi.org/10.1016/j.jaip.2013.06.010.
18. Atkin K, Ahmed W. Living a 'normal' life: young people coping with thalassemia major or sickle cell disorder. Soc Sci Med. 2001;53(5):615–26.
19. Gabe J, Bury M, Ramsay R. Living with asthma: the experiences of young people at home and at school. Soc Sci Med. 2002;55(9):1619–33. https://doi.org/10.1016/S0277-9536(01)00295-7.
20. Guell C. Painful childhood: children living with juvenile arthritis. Qual Health Res. 2007;17(7):884–92. https://doi.org/10.1177/1049732307305883.
21. Heaton J, Raisanen U, Salinas M. 'Rule your condition, don't let it rule you': young adults' sense of mastery in their accounts of growing up with a chronic illness. Sociol Health Illn. 2016;38(1):3–20. https://doi.org/10.1111/1467-9566.12298.
22. Monaghan L, Gabe J. Embodying health identities: a study of young people with asthma. Soc Sci Med. 2016;160:1–8. https://doi.org/10.1016/j.socscimed.2016.05.013.
23. Secor-Turner M, Scal P, Garwick A, Horvath K, Wells CK. Living with juvenile arthritis: adolescents' challenges and experiences. J Pediatr Health Care. 2011;25(5):302–17. https://doi.org/10.1016/j.pedhc.2010.06.004.
24. Lambert V, Keogh D. Striving to live a normal life: a review of children and young people's experience of feeling different when living with a long-term condition. J Pediatr Nurs. 2015;30:63–77. https://doi.org/10.1016/j.pedn.2014.09.016.
25. Taylor RM, Gibson F, Franck LS. The experience of living with a chronic illness during adolescence: a critical review of the literature. J Clin Nurs. 2008;17(23):3083–91. https://doi.org/10.1111/j.1365-2702.2008.02629.x.
26. Tong A, Jones J, Craig JC, Singh-Grewal D. Children's experiences of living with juvenile idiopathic arthritis: a thematic synthesis of qualitative studies. Arthritis Care Res. 2012;64(9):1392–404. https://doi.org/10.1002/acr.21695.
27. Venning A, Eliott J, Wilson A, Kettler L. Understanding young peoples' experience of chronic illness: a systematic review. Int J Evid Based Healthc. 2008;6(3):321–36. https://doi.org/10.1111/j.1744-1609.2008.00107.x.
28. Williams B, Corlett J, Dowell J, Coyle J, Mukhopadhyay S. 'I've never not had it so I don't really know what it's like not to': nondifference and biographical disruption among children and young people with cystic fibrosis. Qual Health Res. 2009;19(10):1443–55. https://doi.org/10.1177/1049732309348363.
29. Barned C, Stinzi A, Mack D, O'Doherty KC. To tell or not to tell: a qualitative interview study on disclosure decisions among children with inflammatory bowel disease. Soc Sci Med. 2016;162:115–23. https://doi.org/10.1016/j.socscimed.2016.06.023.
30. Benson A, Lambert V, Gallagher P, Shahwan A, Austin JK. "I don't want them to look at me and think of my illness, I just want them to look at me and see me": child perspectives on the challenges associated with disclosing an epilepsy diagnosis to others. Epilepsy Behav. 2015;53:83–91. https://doi.org/10.1016/j.yebeh.2015.09.026.
31. Mathur R, Berndt TJ. Relations of friends' activities to friendship quality. J Early Adolesc. 2006;26(3):365–88. https://doi.org/10.1177/0272431606288553.
32. Mellanby AR, Rees JB, Tripp JH. Peer-led and adult-led school health education: a critical review of available comparative research. Health Educ Res. 2000;15(5):533–45. https://doi.org/10.1093/her/15.5.533.
33. Dennis CL. Peer support within a health care context: a concept analysis. Int J Nurs Stud. 2003;40(3):321–32. https://doi.org/10.1016/S0020-7489(02)00092-5.
34. Zhong C, Melendez-Torres GJ. The effect of peer-led self-management education programmes for adolescents with asthma: a systematic review and meta-analysis. Health Educ J. 2017;76(6):676–94. https://doi.org/10.1177/0017896917712297.

35. Eskicioglu P, Halas J, Sénéchal M, Wood L, McKay E, Villeneuve S, Shen GX, Dean H, McGavock JM. Peer mentoring for type 2 diabetes prevention in first nations children. Pediatrics. 2014;133:e1624. https://doi.org/10.1542/peds.2013-2621.
36. Mezey G, Meyer D, Robinson F, Bonell C, Campbell R, Gillard S, Jordan P, Mantovani N, Wellings K, White S. Developing and piloting a peer mentoring intervention to reduce teenage pregnancy in looked-after children and care leavers: an exploratory randomised controlled trial. Health Technol Assess. 2015;19(85):1–509. https://doi.org/10.3310/hta19850.
37. Ali K, Farrer L, Gulliver A, Griffiths K. Online peer-to-peer support for young people with mental health problems: a systematic review. JMIR MHealth. 2015;2(2):e19. https://doi.org/10.2196/mental.4418.
38. Coleman N, Sykes W, Groom C. Peer support and children and young people's mental health research review. London: Department for Education; 2017.
39. Kendal S, Kirk S, Elvey R, Catchpole R, Pryjmachuk S. How a moderated online discussion forum facilitates support for young people with eating disorder. Health Expect. 2016;20(1):98–111. https://doi.org/10.1111/hex.12439.
40. Cassiani C, Stinson J, Lindsay S. E-mentoring for youth with physical disabilities preparing for employment: a content analysis of support exchanged between participants of a mentored and non-mentored group. Disabil Rehabil. 2019;14:1–8. https://doi.org/10.1080/09638288.2018.1543360.
41. Kramer JM, Ryan CT, Moore R, Schwartz A. Feasibility of electronic peer mentoring for transition-age youth and young adults with intellectual and developmental disabilities: project TEAM (Teens making Environment and Activity Modifications). J Appl Res Intellect Disabil. 2018;31(1):e118–29. https://doi.org/10.1111/jar.12346.
42. Lasanen M, Määttä K, Uusiautti S. 'I am not alone' – an ethnographic research on the peer support among northern-Finnish children with hearing loss. Early Child Dev Care. 2019;189(7):1203–18. https://doi.org/10.1080/03004430.2017.1371704.
43. Lindsay S, Hartman LR, Fellin M. A systematic review of mentorship programs to facilitate transition to post-secondary education and employment for youth and young adults with disabilities. Disabil Rehabil. 2016;38(14):1329–49. https://doi.org/10.3109/09638288.2015.1092174.
44. Rhee H, Belyea MJ, Hunt JF, Brasch J. Effects of a peer-led asthma self-management program for adolescents. Arch Pediatr Adolesc Med. 2011;165(6):513–9. https://doi.org/10.1001/archpediatrics.2011.79.
45. Stinson J, Ahola Kohut S, Forgeron P, Amaria A, Bell M, Kaufman M, Luca N, Luca S, Harris L, Victor C, Spiegel L. The iPeer2Peer Program: a pilot randomized controlled trial in adolescents with juvenile idiopathic arthritis. Pediatr Rheumatol. 2016;14(1):48. https://doi.org/10.1186/s12969-016-0108-2.
46. Oris L, Seiffge-Krenke I, Moons P, Goubert L, Rassart J, Goossens E, Luyckx K. Parental and peer support in adolescents with a chronic condition: a typological approach and developmental implications. J Behav Med. 2016;39(1):107–19. https://doi.org/10.1007/s10865-015-9680-z.
47. Shroff Pendley J, Kasmen L, Miller D, Nonze J. Peer and family support in children and adolescents with type 1 diabetes. J Pediatr Psychol. 2002;27(5):429–38. https://doi.org/10.1093/jpepsy/27.5.429.
48. Pittman AF. Implications of peer pressure for adolescent nursing research: a concept analysis approach. Comprehens Child Adolesc Nurs. 2019;42(1):54–70. https://doi.org/10.1080/24694193.2017.1387829.
49. Ahola Kohut S, Stinson J, Forgeron P, van Wyk M, Harris L, Luca S. A qualitative content analysis of peer mentoring video calls in adolescents with chronic illness. J Health Psychol. 2018;23(6):788–99. https://doi.org/10.1177/1359105316669877.
50. Ellis WE, Zarbatany L. Understanding processes of peer clique influence in late childhood and early adolescence. Child Dev Perspect. 2017;11(4):227–32. https://doi.org/10.1111/cdep.12248.

51. Schunk D, Meece J. Self-efficacy development in adolescence. In: Pajares F, Urdan T, editors. Self-efficacy beliefs of adolescents. Greenwich, CT: Information Age Publishing; 2006. p. 71–96.
52. Grape A, Rhee H, Sanchez P. Evaluation of a peer-led asthma self-management group intervention for urban adolescents. J Pediatr Nurs. 2019;45:1–6. https://doi.org/10.1016/j. pedn.2018.12.011.
53. Nabors L, Ige TJ, Fevrier B. Peer support and psychosocial pain management strategies for children with systemic lupus erythematosus. J Immunol Res. 2015;2015:238263. https://doi. org/10.1155/2015/238263.
54. Birks Y, Sloper P, Lewin R, Parsons J. Exploring health-related experiences of children and young people with congenital heart disease. Health Expect. 2007;10(1):16–29. https://doi. org/10.1111/j.1369-7625.2006.00412.x.
55. LaGreca A, Bearman K, Moore H. Peer relations of youth with pediatric conditions and health risks: promoting social support and healthy lifestyles. J Dev Behav Pediatr. 2002;2(23):271–80. https://doi.org/10.1097/00004703-200208000-00013.
56. Sattoe JNT, Jedeloo S, van Staa AL. Effective peer-to-peer support for young people with end-stage renal disease: a mixed methods evaluation of Camp COOL. BMC Nephrol. 2013;14:279. https://doi.org/10.1186/1471-2369-14-279.
57. Stewart M, Letourneau N, Masuda JR, Anderson S, McGhan S. Impacts of online peer support for children with asthma and allergies: "it just helps you every time you can't breathe well". J Pediatr Nurs. 2013;28(5):439–52. https://doi.org/10.1016/j.pedn.2013.01.003.
58. Kirk S, Hinton D. "I'm not what I used to be": a qualitative study exploring how young people experience being diagnosed with a chronic illness. Child Care Health Dev. 2019;45(2):216–26. https://doi.org/10.1111/cch.12638.
59. Kaushansky D, Cox J, Dodson C, McNeeley M, Kumar S, Iverson E. Living a secret: disclosure among adolescents and young adults with chronic illnesses. Chronic Illn. 2017;13(1):49–61. https://doi.org/10.1177/1742395316655855.
60. Pini S, Gardner P, Hugh-Jones S. What effect does a cancer diagnosis have on the educational engagement and school life of teenagers? A systematic review. Psychooncology. 2012;21(7):685–94. https://doi.org/10.1002/pon.2082.
61. D'Auria JP, Christian B, Henderson Z, Haynes B. The company they keep: the influence of peer relationships on adjustment to cystic fibrosis during adolescence. J Pediatr Nurs. 2000;15(3):175–82. https://doi.org/10.1053/jn.2000.6023.
62. Kirk S, Beatty S, Callery P, Milnes L, Pryjmachuk S. Perceptions of effective self-care support for children and young people with long-term conditions. J Clin Nurs. 2012;21(13–14):1974–87. https://doi.org/10.1111/j.1365-2702.2011.04027.x.
63. Oxford English Dictionary. Oxford English Dictionary online. 2019. https://www.oed.com/.
64. Sandhu S, Veinot P, Embuldeniya G, Brooks S, Sale J, Huang S, Zhao A, Richards D, Bell MJ. Peer to-peer mentoring for individuals with early inflammatory arthritis: feasibility pilot. BMJ Open. 2013;3:e002267. https://doi.org/10.1136/bmjopen-2012-002267.
65. Repper J, Carter T. A review of the literature on peer support in mental health services. J Ment Health. 2011;20(4):392–411. https://doi.org/10.3109/09638237.2011.583947.
66. Breakey VR, Bouskill V, Nguyen C, Lucas S, Stinson J, Ahola Kohut S. Online peer-to-peer mentoring support for youth with hemophilia: qualitative needs assessment. JMIR Pediatr Parent. 2018;1(2):e10958. https://doi.org/10.2196/10958.
67. Munce SEP, Shepherd J, Perrier L, Allin S, Sweet S, Tomasone JR, Nelson M, Guilcher S, Hossain S, Jaglal S. Online peer support interventions for chronic conditions: a scoping review protocol. BMJ Open. 2017;7:e017999. https://doi.org/10.1136/bmjopen-2017-017999.
68. Bennett PN, St. Clair Russell J, Atwal J, Brown L, Schiller B. Patient-to-patient peer mentor support in dialysis: improving the patient experience. Semin Dial. 2018;31(5):455–61. https://doi.org/10.1111/sdi.12703.
69. Fortuna KL, Brooks JM, Umucu E, Walker R, Chow PI. Peer support: a human factor to enhance engagement in digital health behavior change interventions. J Technol Behav Sci. 2019;4(2):152. https://doi.org/10.1007/s41347-019-00105-x.

70. Mead S, MacNeil C. Peer support: what makes it unique. Int J Psychosoc Rehabil. 2006;10(2):29–37.
71. Lewis P, Klineberg E, Towns S, Moore K, Steinbeck K. The effects of introducing peer support to young people with a chronic illness. J Child Fam Stud. 2016;25:2541–53. https://doi.org/10.1007/s10826-016-0427-4.
72. Lazarus RS, Folkman S. Stress, appraisal, and coping. New York, NY: Springer; 1984.
73. Bandura A, Ramachaudran VS. Encyclopedia of human behavior. New York, NY: Academic Press; 1994.
74. Sarason IG, Levine HM, Basham RB, Sarason BR. Assessing social support: the social support questionnaire. J Pers Soc Psychol. 1983;44(1):127–39. https://doi.org/10.1037/0022-3514.44.1.127.
75. Mead S, Hilton D, Curtis L. Peer support: a theoretical perspective. Psychiatr Rehabil J. 2001;25(2):134–41. https://doi.org/10.1037/h0095032.
76. Bal MI, Sattoe JNT, Roelofs PD, Bal R, van Staa AL, Miedema HS. Exploring effectiveness and effective components of self-management interventions for young people with chronic physical conditions: a systematic review. Patient Educ Couns. 2016;99(8):1293–309. https://doi.org/10.1016/j.pec.2016.02.012.
77. Kirk S, Beatty S, Callery P, Gellatly J, Milnes L, Pryjmachuk S. The effectiveness of self-care support interventions for children and young people with long-term conditions: a systematic review. Child Care Health Dev. 2013;39(3):305–24. https://doi.org/10.1111/j.1365-2214.2012.01395.x.
78. Sattoe JNT, Bal MI, Roelofs PD, Bal R, Miedema HS, van Staa AL. Self-management interventions for young people with chronic conditions: a systematic overview. Patient Educ Couns. 2015;98(6):704–15. https://doi.org/10.1016/j.pec.2015.03.004.
79. Stenberg U, Haaland-Øverby M, Koricho AT, Trollvik A, Kristoffersen LR, Dybvig S, Vågan A. How can we support children, adolescents and young adults in managing chronic health challenges? A scoping review on the effects of patient education interventions. Health Expect. 2019;22(5):849–62. https://doi.org/10.1111/hex.12906.
80. Christian BJ, D'Auria JP. Building life skills for children with cystic fibrosis: effectiveness of an intervention. Nurs Res. 2006;55(5):300–7. https://doi.org/10.1097/00006199-200609000-00002.
81. Békési A, Török S, Kökönyei G, Bokrétás I, Szentes A, Telepóczki G, The European KIDSCREEN Group. Health-related quality of life changes of children and adolescents with chronic disease after participation in therapeutic recreation camping program. Health Qual Life Outcomes. 2011;9:43. https://doi.org/10.1186/1477-7525-9-43.
82. Moola FJ, Faulkner GE, White L, Kirsh JA. The psychological and social impact of camp for children with chronic illnesses: a systematic review update. Child Care Health Dev. 2013;40(5):615–31. https://doi.org/10.1111/cch.12114.
83. Desai PP, Sutton LJ, Staley MD, Hannon DW. A qualitative study exploring the psychosocial value of weekend camping experiences for children and adolescents with complex heart defects. Child Care Health Dev. 2013;40(4):553–61. https://doi.org/10.1111/cch.12056.
84. Gillard A, Witt PA, Watts CE. Outcomes and processes at a camp for youth with HIV/AIDS. Qual Health Res. 2011;21(11):1508–26. https://doi.org/10.1177/1049732311413907.
85. Gillard A, Allsop J. Camp experiences in the lives of adolescents with serious illnesses. Children Youth Serv Rev. 2016;65:112–9. https://doi.org/10.1016/j.childyouth.2016.04.001.
86. Hackett J, Johnson B, Shaw KL, McDonagh JE. Friends united: an evaluation of an innovative residential self-management programme in adolescent rheumatology. Br J Occup Ther. 2005;68(12):567–73. https://doi.org/10.1177/030802260506801206.
87. Kiernan G, Gormley M, MacLachlan M. Outcomes associated with participation in a therapeutic recreation camping programme for children from 15 European countries: data from the 'Barretstown Studies'. Soc Sci Med. 2004;59(5):903–13. https://doi.org/10.1016/j.socscimed.2003.12.010.
88. Kiernan G, Guerin S, MacLachlan M. Children's voices: qualitative data from the 'Barretstown studies'. Int J Nurs Stud. 2005;42(7):733–41. https://doi.org/10.1016/j.ijnurstu.2003.05.003.

89. Al-Sheyab N, Gallagher R, Crisp J, Shah S. Peer-led education for adolescents with asthma in Jordan: a cluster-randomized controlled trial. Pediatrics. 2012;129(1):e106–12. https://doi.org/10.1542/peds.2011-0346.

90. Gibson PG, Shah S, Mamoon HA. Peer-led asthma education for adolescents: impact evaluation. J Adolesc Health. 1998;22:66–72. https://doi.org/10.1016/S1054-139X(97)00203-6.

91. Shah S, Peat JK, Mazurski EJ, Wang H, Sindhusake D, Bruce C, Henry RL, Gibson PG. Effect of peer led programme for asthma education in adolescents: cluster randomised controlled trial. Br Med J. 2001;322(7286):583–5. https://doi.org/10.1136/bmj.322.7286.583.

92. Salinas M. Evaluation study of the staying positive pilot workshops: a self-management programme for young people with chronic conditions. Oxford: Department of Public Health, University of Oxford; 2007.

93. Løding RN, Wold JE, Skavhaug A, Graue M. Evaluation of peer-group support and problem-solving training in the treatment of adolescents with type 1 diabetes. Eur Diabetes Nurs. 2007;4(1):28–33. https://doi.org/10.1002/edn.73.

94. Scheel A, Beatona A, Okellob E, Longenecker CT, Otim I, Lwabi P, Sable C, Webel A, Aliku T. The impact of a peer support group for children with rheumatic heart disease in Uganda. Patient Educ Couns. 2018;101(1):119–23. https://doi.org/10.1016/j.pec.2017.07.006.

95. Naar-King S, Outlaw A, Green-Jones M, Wright K, Parsons JT. Motivational interviewing by peer outreach workers: a pilot randomized clinical trial to retain adolescents and young adults in HIV care. AIDS Care. 2009;21(7):868–73. https://doi.org/10.1080/09540120802612824.

96. Jerson B, D'urso C, Arnon R, Miloh T, Iyer K, Kerkar N, Annunziato RA. Adolescent transplant recipients as peer mentors: a program to improve self-management and health-related quality of life. Pediatr Transplant. 2013;17(7):612–20. https://doi.org/10.1111/petr.12127.

97. Cassano J, Nagel K, O'Mara L. Talking with others who "just know": perceptions of adolescents with cancer who participate in a teen group. J Pediatr Oncol Nurs. 2008;25(4):193–9. https://doi.org/10.1177/1043454208319972.

98. Olsson CA, Boyce MF, Toumbourou JW, Sawyer SM. The role of peer support in facilitating psychosocial adjustment to chronic illness in adolescence. Clin Child Psychol Psychiatry. 2005;10:78–87. https://doi.org/10.1177/1359104505048793.

99. Ahola Kohut S, Stinson J, Forgeron P, Luca S, Harris L. Been there, done that: the experience of acting as a young adult mentor to adolescents living with chronic illness. J Pediatr Psychol. 2017;42(9):962–9. https://doi.org/10.1093/jpepsy/jsx062.

100. Letourneau N, Stewart M, Masuda JR, Anderson S, Cicutto L, McGhan S, Watt S. Impact of online support for youth with asthma and allergies: pilot study. J Pediatr Nurs. 2012;27:65–73. https://doi.org/10.1016/j.pedn.2010.07.007.

101. Masuda JR, Anderson S, Letourneau N, Morgan VS, Stewart M. Reconciling preferences and constraints in online peer support for youth with asthma and allergies. Health Promot Pract. 2013;14(5):741–50. https://doi.org/10.1177/1524839912465083.

102. Johnson KB, Ravery RD, Everton A. Hopkins Teen Central: assessment of an internet-based support system for children with cystic fibrosis. Pediatrics. 2001;107:e24. https://doi.org/10.1542/peds.107.2.e24.

103. Nicholas DB, Picone G, Vigneux A, McCormick K, Mantulak A, McClure M, Macculloch R. Evaluation of an online peer support network for adolescents with chronic kidney disease. J Technol Hum Serv. 2009;27:23–33. https://doi.org/10.1080/15228830802462063.

104. Kirk S, Milnes L. An exploration of how young people and parents use online support in the context of living with cystic fibrosis. Health Expect. 2016;19(2):309–21. https://doi.org/10.1111/hex.12352.

105. Ravert RD, Hancock MD, Ingersoll GM. Online forum messages posted by adolescents with type 1 diabetes. Diabetes Educ. 2004;30(5):827–34. https://doi.org/10.1177/014572170403000518.

106. Husted GR, Weis J, Teilmann G, Castensøe-Seidenfaden P. Exploring the influence of a smartphone app (young with diabetes) on young people's self-management: qualitative study. JMIR Mhealth. 2018;6(2):e43. https://doi.org/10.2196/mhealth.8876.

107. Epstein I, Stinson J, Stevens B. The effects of camp on health-related quality of life in children with chronic illnesses: a review of the literature. J Pediatr Oncol Nurs. 2005;22:89–103. https://doi.org/10.1177/1043454204273881.
108. Rhee H, McQuillan BE, Belyea MJ. Evaluation of a peer-led asthma self-management program and benefits of the program for adolescent peer leaders. Respiratory care. 2012a; 57(12):2082–9.
109. Rhee H, Pesis-Katz I, Xing J. Cost benefits of a peer-led asthma self-management program for adolescents. J Asthma. 2012b;49(6):606–13. https://doi.org/10.3109/02770903.2012. 694540.
110. Merianos AL, King KA, Vidourek RA, Nabors LA. Mentoring and peer-led interventions to improve quality of life outcomes among adolescents with chronic illnesses. Appl Res Qual Life. 2016;11:1009–23. https://doi.org/10.1007/s11482-015-9415-x.
111. Sansom-Daly RM, Peate M, Wakefield CE, Bryant R, Cohn R. A systematic review of psychological interventions for adolescents and young adults living with chronic illness. Health Psychol. 2012;31(3):380–93. https://doi.org/10.1037/a0025977.
112. Waite-Jones J, Swallow V. Peer-based social support for young-people with juvenile arthritis: views of young people, parents/carers and healthcare professionals within the UK. J Pediatr Nurs. 2018;43:e85–91. https://doi.org/10.1016/j.pedn.2018.07.012.
113. Nesta. People helping people: peer support that changes lives. London: Nesta; 2013.
114. NHS England, Care Quality Commission, Health Education England, Monitor, Public Health England, & Trust Development Authority. NHS five year forward view. London: NHS England; 2014.
115. NHS. The NHS long term plan. London: NHS England; 2019.
116. Nesta & National Voices. Peer support: what is it and does it work. London: National Voices; 2015.
117. Cambridge & Peterborough NHS Foundation Trust. Recovery. 2020. https://www.cpft.nhs. uk/patients/peer-support.htm.
118. Backett-Milburn K, Wilson S. Understanding peer education: insights from a process evaluation. Health Educ Res. 2000;15(1):85–96.
119. Larsson I, Staland-Nyman C, Svedberg P, Nygren JM, Carlson I. Children and young people's participation in developing interventions in health and well-being: a scoping review. BMC Health Serv Res. 2018;18:507. https://doi.org/10.1186/s12913-018-3219-2.
120. Medical Research Council. Developing and evaluating complex interventions. London: Medical Research Council; 2006.

Skills for Growing Up and Ready Steady Go: Practical Tools to Promote Life Skills in Youth with Chronic Conditions

Jane N. T. Sattoe, AnneLoes van Staa, Marij E. Roebroeck, and Sander R. Hilberink

8.1   Introduction

Youth with chronic conditions face the same challenges on their way to adulthood as their typical developing peers but encounter additional bumps in the road because of their chronic condition and its consequences. Becoming an adult—the transition into adulthood—requires the mastery of life skills (i.e. being able to perform adult roles). This transition occurs in several life areas, such as education and employment, interpersonal relationships and sexuality, finances and housing. As Binks et al. [1] noted, transition should be considered as a process rather than an event, and therefore each adolescent should be timely prepared for future roles. In fact, transition into adulthood ideally is a gradual shift, consisting of several steps to acquire age-appropriate life skills.

The importance of preparing youth for future roles requires a future-oriented approach in healthcare. Next to paying attention to symptoms and the treatment of the chronic condition, healthcare professionals need to tune to the specific developmental phase the young person goes through (see Chap. 5). This implies that addressing the development of autonomy and social participation (e.g. relationships with peers, education and leisure) becomes increasingly important for youth. Moreover, because the chronic condition impacts their development of autonomy and their opportunities to participate [2], young people with chronic conditions are at risk for overprotection by their parents [3, 4]. While young people with chronic conditions

J. N. T. Sattoe (✉) · A. van Staa · S. R. Hilberink
Research Center Innovations in Care, Rotterdam University of Applied Sciences,
Rotterdam, The Netherlands
e-mail: j.n.t.sattoe@hr.nl

M. E. Roebroeck
Department of Rehabilitation Medicine, Erasmus MC University Medical Center and
Rijndam Rehabilitation, Rotterdam, The Netherlands

© Springer Nature Switzerland AG 2021
J. N. T. Sattoe et al. (eds.), *Self-Management of Young People with Chronic Conditions*, https://doi.org/10.1007/978-3-030-64293-8_8

repeatedly stress the importance to discuss their future roles in the various life areas during healthcare consultations, these topics are often underexposed [3, 5, 6].

To open up discussions about developmental tasks and challenges during healthcare consultations, the use of comprehensive individual transition plans has been advocated [6–8]. Such plans help to regularly monitor the development of autonomy of youth in various life areas. Unlike transition readiness assessments that are more focused on medical management (e.g. disease knowledge) and assessment of treatment-related skills [9], individual transition plans are helpful to monitor the development of independence and autonomy, and as such can provide guidelines for action for young people, their parents and healthcare professionals. In this chapter, we discuss two specific examples of transition plans that facilitate the communication about the development of age-appropriate life skills from childhood to late-adolescence: the Skills for Growing Up (SGU) and the Ready Steady Go (RSG) tools. Since the developmental challenges are similar across chronic conditions, these tools are generic and can be used for all young people. The SGU, however, has diagnosis-specific adjustments. We elaborate on the theoretical framework, the content and structure of, and the first experiences with, and outcomes of these tools.

8.2   Theoretical Framework

The underlying concepts of both tools stem from the Basic Psychological Needs Theory, part of the Self-Determination Theory [10, 11], although not specifically mentioned by the developers. According to these, having autonomy, competence and relatedness are fundamental psychological human needs. In the Self-Determination Theory, autonomy refers to behaviour based on willpower and choice; competence refers to being able to master the environment; and relatedness means being connected with other persons in social constructs. In addition, having autonomy is essential for healthy functioning [12], and is a prerequisite for developing oneself as a motivated agent. It is important to distinguish between *executional autonomy* (being able to self-perform) and *decisional autonomy* (being able to make own choices) [13]. These principles are reflected in both the SGU and RSG. Both tools aim to support the development of competences (e.g. life skills). Youth are encouraged to take the lead, they are challenged to do certain things themselves (e.g. making a meal) or, if they cannot *do* it because of the disability or chronic condition, to take charge of it (e.g. deciding what has to be cooked). Relatedness is supported by addressing the importance of finding support when needed, developing friendships, intimacy and sexuality.

Although the development of autonomy is an ongoing process that onsets at a very young age, children need to have certain cognitive abilities to explicitly develop autonomy and reflect on it. Hence, the SGU can be used by children of 7 years or older, whereas the RSG is appropriate for youth of 12 years and older. Autonomy and acquiring competences are also corner stones in the Positive Youth Development (PYD) perspective [14] (see Chap. 2). PYD interventions focus on positive outcomes (i.e. self-advocacy, skill building and relationships with others). Both tools presented in this chapter can be seen as PYD-approaches because these support

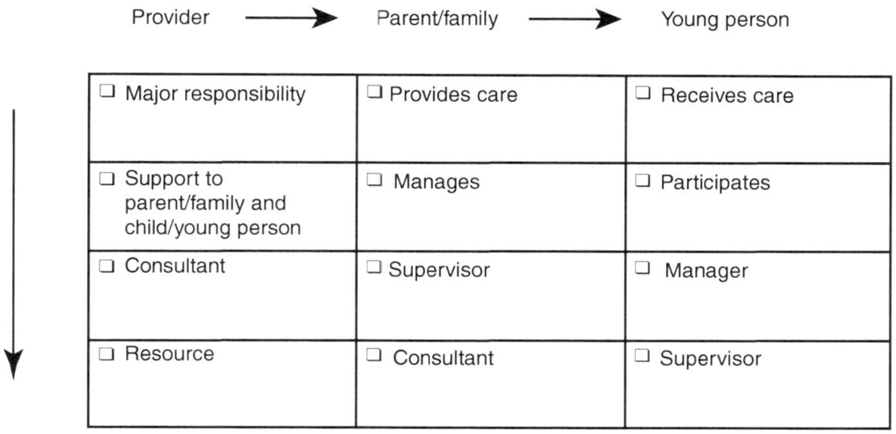

| Provider | ⟶ | Parent/family | ⟶ | Young person |

❏ Major responsibility	❏ Provides care	❏ Receives care
❏ Support to parent/family and child/young person	❏ Manages	❏ Participates
❏ Consultant	❏ Supervisor	❏ Manager
❏ Resource	❏ Consultant	❏ Supervisor

Fig. 8.1 Shared management model. (Growing Up Ready, Carie Gall, Shauna Kingsnorth, et al., Physical and Occupational Therapy in Pediatrics, 2006, reprinted with permission of Taylor & Francis Ltd, http://www.tandfonline.com)

normal development and promote the development of life skills. Also, both tools follow the framework of the Shared Management Model (SMM) [15]. The SMM outlines the gradual shift in responsibility for health, care and functioning from parents or caregivers to the child as he/she grows older (Fig. 8.1). The SGU and RSG align with this by proposing a stepwise approach to the development of competencies of youth across different ages.

8.3   Skills for Growing Up

The SGU approach was developed in Canada (Holland Bloorview Kids Rehabilitation Hospital) and was adapted for use in Dutch paediatric rehabilitation care (SGU-Dutch) [16, 17], paediatric nephrology (SGU-Nephrology) [18] and paediatric epilepsy care (SGU-Epilepsy) [3]. The tool is based on four key principles: (1) universality (encouraging family interaction about age-appropriate development), (2) family centredness, (3) shared management and (4) developmental approach [19].

The SGU consists of three (developmental) age-appropriate item lists: 'Getting started' (7–11 years), 'On my way' (12–16 years) and 'Almost there' (17 years or older). Additionally, there is a list for parents (not for the SGU-Dutch). Each item list in the Dutch version covers nine life areas: Me, Healthcare, Living and ADL (activities of daily living), Relationships, Education, Transportation, Sports, Leisure activities, and Employment (Fig. 8.2). All life areas contain items that represent age-appropriate knowledge, skills or activities per area (see Box 8.1). Per item, a young person can indicate whether he or she already possesses the mentioned knowledge, or skills or already performs the specific activity. Parents fill out whether or not they think their child already knows about the topics raised, masters the mentioned skills, and performs

Fig. 8.2 Life areas in the SGU. (With permission from: Hilberink et al. (2020). Focus on autonomy: Using 'Skills for Growing Up' in pediatric rehabilitation care. Journal of Pediatric Rehabilitation Medicine, 13, 161–167)

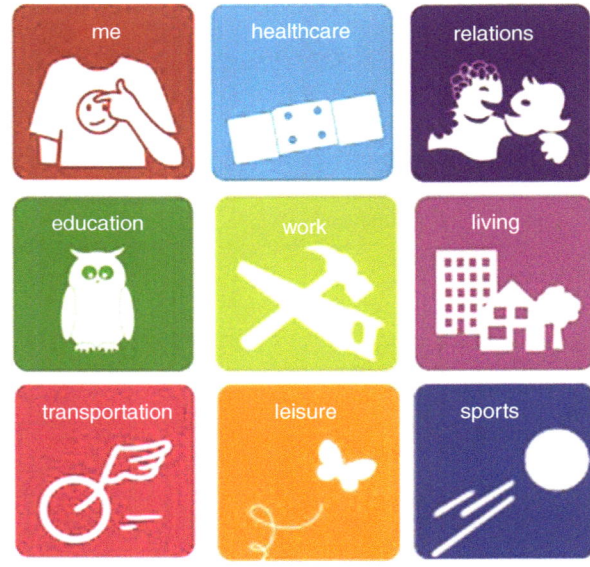

Box 8.1: Item Examples and Action Plan Format of the Skills for Growing Up Tool[a]

Me

   'I can tell others what my condition is and what it practically means for my daily life' (12–16 years)

    Healthcare

    'I know what to do when I forget to take my medication' (12–16 years)

    Relationships

    'I spend time with my friends outside school' (12–16 years)

    Education

    'I know what to do to get an internship' (17+ years)

    Work

    'I know the influence of my condition on work' (17+ years)

    Living and ADL

    'I sometimes do chores at home' (7–11 years)

    Transportation

    'I travel by myself by public transportation' (17+ years)

    Leisure activities

    'I attend a camp, like school camp or soccer camp' (7–11 years)

    Sports

    'I can swim' (7–11 years)

    Action plan

Step 1: I want to work on the following items:
[items scored with no]
Step 2: I will take the following steps to work on these items:
[description of steps to take]
Step 3: I will work on these items on:
[description of step] [date]
[a]Republished with permission of Sattoe et al. 2014 [18]

the tasks or activities independently. At the end of the list, youth can choose which items they would like to work on for the coming period and are stimulated to make an action plan accordingly. They can also write down any questions they have. The lists and action plans are discussed during consultations with healthcare professionals.

While the aforementioned SGUs are developed for youth with normal intelligence, youth (with or without epilepsy) with a mild intellectual disability can use the SGU-ID (intellectual disability). The SGU-ID has two age-appropriate item lists: 'Getting started' (7–13 years) and 'Almost there' (14 years or older). These lists consist of fewer items and items are phrased vernacular compared to the other SGU tools. Rotterdam University of Applied Sciences and Rijndam Rehabilitation provide the Dutch SGU lists for free at: https://www.opeigenbenen.nu/professionals/transitie-toolkit/tool_groei-wijzer/, and at: https://www.rijndam.nl/innovatie-onderzoek/productcatalogus-voor-zorgprofessionals/e-learning-hoe-werk-ik-met-de-groei. An e-learning has been developed to support professionals in child rehabilitation in using the SGU-Dutch https://www.free-learning.nl/modules/groei-wijzer-in-derevalidatie/start.html.

The SGU tools aim to encourage the communication about the development of autonomy and life skills between youths and parents and between youths, parents and the healthcare professionals. In other words, it aims to hold up a mirror to show what constitutes 'typical' age-appropriate development and to make a stepwise action plan according to the chosen life skills. Therefore, the SGU is not a checklist to measure ones 'life skills' status', but rather a communication tool to promote discussion about autonomy and empowerment of youth with chronic conditions. In Box 8.2 an illustrative case of a consultation with a boy and his mother is presented.

Box 8.2: Application of the Skills for Growing Up Tool: An Example
A few days ago, Eli and his parents came to the children's rehabilitation centre for consultation. Recently, he turned 18 years old and he is planning on pursuing further education. He will be transferred to adult rehabilitation soon. Before the consultation, both Eli and his mother filled out the Skills for Growing Up lists. In the past few years in rehabilitation care, attention has been given to Eli's development of independence and autonomy, but the therapists felt that Eli has not been able to show his potential. They gave him and his parents the Skills for Growing Up lists to facilitate interaction between them about his

development. Eli filled out the list together with his mom and came up with some points he would like to work on. During consultation, the therapist asked him about this, but before Eli could respond his mother took over. Quickly the conversation evolved between his mother and the therapist and was *about* Eli instead of *with* him. Eli's mother for instance complained about him sleeping way past breakfast time in the weekends, and about him being busy on his phone all the time. The therapist noticed that Eli was not feeling comfortable to say anything and turned the conversation. He explained that things that parents see as problems are not always problems for their children. Actually, wasn't Eli's behaviour appropriate for his age? After this was clear, the conversation about Eli's future could start. The therapist asked him again and Eli told him that he would like to live independently after finishing his vocational education. He said the Skills for Growing Up lists encouraged him think about what would be needed for him to live independently and how he could take the lead. He, for example, mentioned that he could make his own breakfast instead of waiting for his mother. Together with the therapist Eli developed an action plan to work on his independency in household activities, starting with making his own meals. He actively thought about the right time to start doing this and about who he could ask for help if needed. This conversation made his mother aware of amount of help she and her husband offered Eli. She admitted that Eli's behaviour was common for his age and that he should get more room to try to do things. Instead of his parents solving everything for him, Eli should be encouraged and facilitated to take care of himself. For Eli's parents, the consultation with the Skills for Growing Up list helped them to put the choices and wishes of Eli before their own. For Eli, the consultation with the Skills for Growing Up list lead to a conversation about becoming independent and eventually resulted in a tailormade action plan. He became aware of the fact that, while he is not ready to live independently yet, he could take the lead in working towards independency in small steps. He is the one who has to take action, but he can always ask for help if needed.

8.4   Ready Steady Go

The RSG tool was originally developed in the United Kingdom and is a continuation of previously developed individual transition plans for young people with rheumatoid arthritis [20]. It has been translated into French, Spanish, Dutch, Portuguese, Thai and Japanese [21]. The tool aims to prepare youth for the transfer to adult care, to support the development of autonomy, and to empower youth in order to improve long-term outcomes [22]. Although not explicitly mentioned as an aim of the RSG, some introduce the tool as a way to improve therapeutic adherence [21]. In contrast to the SGU, the RSG has not been not adjusted for specific diagnose groups and should be considered as a generic tool that can be used across different chronic conditions.

The RSG consists of four age-appropriate item lists: Ready (11/12–14 years), Steady (14–16 years), Go (16–18 years) and Hello (18–25 years). Each item list used in paediatric care covers eight domains: Knowledge (about the chronic condition and therapy), Self-advocacy (speaking up for yourself), Health and lifestyle, Daily living, School/career/your future, Leisure, Managing your emotions and Transfer do adult care. The list used in adult care (Hello) does not address transfer to adult care anymore and thus has seven domains. Items consider knowledge, skills and activities in the different domains (see Box 8.3). Recently, Easy Read versions of the Ready Steady Go lists have been developed [23].

The working way is the same as for the SGU: youth report per item whether or not they possess the mentioned knowledge, skills or perform the activities. There is, however, an extra column per item asking whether the young person wants to know more about this particular item. At the end of the lists they can write down anything else they wish to discuss with their healthcare provider. The lists are discussed during consultations with healthcare professionals. Youth are also encouraged to make an action plan, although this is not specifically mentioned on the RSG lists. If preferred, they could do so in collaboration with parents and/or healthcare providers during consultations. The University Hospital Southamptom/NHS provides the original RSG materials for free: http://www.uhs.nhs.uk/OurServices/Childhealth/TransitiontoadultcareReadySteadyGo/Transitiontoadultcare.aspx. Rotterdam University of Applied Sciences also provides the Dutch RSG materials for free at: https://www.opeigenbenen.nu/professionals/transitie-toolkit/tool_ready-steady-go/. The RSG tool is, just like the SGU, a communication tool to foster empowerment and autonomy in young people with chronic conditions, not a questionnaire to measure transition readiness.

Box 8.3: Item Examples of the Ready Steady Go Tool
Knowledge
  'I am confident in my knowledge about my condition and its management' (Go)
  Self-advocacy
  'I feel ready to start preparing to be seen alone for part of the clinic visit in the future' (Ready)
  Health and lifestyle
  'I understand the risks of alcohol, drugs and smoking to my health' (Ready)
  Daily living
  'I can make my own snacks/meals' (Steady)
  School/career/your future
  'I am managing at college/work e.g. getting to and around, nature of work, friends etc.' (Hello)
  Leisure
  'I can use public transport and access my local community e.g. shops, leisure centre, cinema' (Hello)
  Managing your emotions
  'I am happy with life' (Go)
  Transfer to adult care
  'I am aware of the plan for my medical care when I am an adult' (Steady)

8.5   Experiences of Youth and Their Parents

Youth and their parents report positive experiences with both tools and mention several benefits of their use. Since these overlap between the RSG and SGU tools, we will discuss them without distinguishing between the specific tools. First, youth and parents agreed with the content of the item lists and in general felt that all life areas or domains in the lists were appropriate and relevant for them [3, 18, 21, 22]. However, a small group of youth in one study doubted the relevancy of the tool and reported that filling out competency lists reminds them of school work and doing exams, which is not a positive thing [3]. Another study found that the value youth attached to the tool correlated with age and youth's self-efficacy. Younger persons and those with lower self-efficacy seemed to appreciate the tool more [17].

Second, young people felt that the tool helped them in communication and inter-action with both their parents and healthcare professionals [3, 16]. It made it possible for them to share their wishes, expectations and what they thought is important. According to healthcare professionals parents also mentioned that the tool sup-ported their interaction with their child [18]. This was also found in another study where parents indicate that the tool made it easier for them to discuss transition-related topics with their children [24].

Third, youth report that use of the tool made them more aware of their independence and future prospects and stimulated them to make conscious efforts to obtain independence from their parents [3, 16]. Parents share the positive note about awareness, although some mentioned that the tool could also be confronting. For example, one parent mentioned that before filling out the item list he or she never thought about the future of his/her child with epilepsy, while he/she did think about the future of his/her other children without epilepsy. The tool was an eye-opener for this parent [3]. The benefit of increased awareness was also mentioned by parents of young people with end-stage kidney disease [18] and by parents of youth treated in rehabilitation care [24]. Finally, youth and their parents in general found both instruments to be supportive tools to develop autonomy and acquire life skills, and to achieve developmental milestones in small steps [16]. For example, young people with type 1 diabetes explicitly appreciated that the steps to independence start at an early age [25].

However, there are also some areas of concern. One study showed that youth with spina bifida following special education, seemed to have more problems with understanding the items and filling out the lists on their own. These young people were also less satisfied with the tool compared to those not following special education [26]. The same was true for youth with significant learning needs in another study [21]. To counter this, perhaps the version for young people with mild intellectual disability (SGU-ID) [27] or the specially developed 'Easy Read' versions of the RSG or the RSG version for use on a tablet [21] can be used. Another critique is that answering in 'yes' or 'no' dichotomy is not always easy. Often 'sometimes' is also the right answer and this might hinder the use of the tool [26], although adding a third answer category could also complicate the use of the tool if young people are more inclined to choose the 'safe' 'sometimes' option.

8.6   Experiences of Healthcare Professionals

Overall, healthcare professionals appreciate the tools and their aims [3, 6, 16–18, 22]. Depending on the setting, the tools are used by different disciplines. In paediatric somatic care, this is most often the (specialized) nurse [3, 18, 21]; in paediatric rehabilitation care, it depends on the local organization: sometimes it is the occupational therapist who uses the tool, in other centres a social worker, psychologist, or special education professionals [16].

Healthcare professionals report different benefits of using individual transition plans such as the RSG and the SGU. The first is that it creates awareness in all parties involved [6, 16, 18]. In professionals, particularly, it helped them to be more focused on the young person (instead of the parent or carer) and to employ a more holistic approach that provides room to discuss difficult topics during healthcare consultations [6, 16, 18]. Professionals treating youth with type 1 diabetes, for instance, experienced that young people experienced a lower threshold to speak up about subjects when using the RSG [25], and professionals working with the SGU-D in paediatric rehabilitation care noticed improved communication with youth [16]. Furthermore, professionals valued that the tool helped them to start raise awareness about autonomy development and self-management from an early age and that it stimulated youth and parents to take small steps in this development [18]. Also, healthcare professionals reported that use of the tools fostered family interaction about development of autonomy and independence [6, 16, 18].

However, in one study professionals also mention a point of attention. Although they all agreed that all life areas included in the SGU-N are important, some felt hesitant to discuss non-medical issues with young people [18]. They were wondering if their roles should extend beyond the medical domain to areas such as living and transportation. Other obstacles both for SGU and RSG relate to implementation and are discussed in the next paragraph.

8.7   Implementation Issues

Although the experiences with both tools are generally positive, the implementation in routine daily care remains a challenge. In case of the RSG, implementation is hampered by the workload of the healthcare teams [21]. Similarly, the use of the SGU-N has been found time-consuming which hindered its use [18]. This has been attributed to the lengthiness of the lists of the SGU-N. Also, professionals did not have enough time to review the lists, because youth and parents did not bring them to consultations [6, 18]. To counter the logistic problems, more user friendly digital forms of the lists, for example an App, would be useful [18], as has also been mentioned for the RSG [21]. Another issue is that it is important keep track of the topics that have been dealt with, which requires maintaining good documentation in the EPR [21]. Some nurses using the tool implemented electronic checklists to do so [6], but there are no standardized ways or recommendations for good documentation of the process.

An important step towards broader implementation of the tools is that their use is recommended in clinical guidelines; for example, the SGU is recommended in the treatment guideline for children with cerebral palsy [28]. Still, it is not always easy to convince professionals to value the more holistic approach and the needed change in healthcare delivery [18, 21]. Professionals questioned whether it is their task to monitor more generic life skills development, and felt that the medical domain is primarily where their tasks lay. Also, traditionally, professionals are used to a more directive role in healthcare, whereas the use of the SGU or RSG asks for a coaching role of professionals. In case of the SGU-N for instance, some professionals regretted that the tool was not supposed to be used as a checklist or an assessment [18]. This is in line with the issue of ownership mentioned by van Staa et al. [6]. They explained that some professionals viewed individual transition plans as something that young people themselves own. They felt the main aim is to empower these young people. Other professionals, however, felt the lists should primarily benefit the healthcare teams.

8.8   Perceived Effectiveness

Studies of the effectiveness of individual transition plans such as the SGU and RSG are scarce. Yet, the few studies that did research the outcomes of these tools, mostly show promising results. Adolescents using the SGU-N for instance, reported a higher frequency of discussions of non-medical topics [6]. In general, youth felt the tools helped them to become more independent, to plan their future and to prepare for their transfer to adult care [6, 16]. For the RSG, Cable and Davis [29] also noted a trend towards more talking about non-medical topics that were found important by young people. Nagra et al. [22] found that professionals had a more holistic approach and that it was easier to address sensitive topics during consultations when the RSG was used. Two studies also found some effects of the RSG on clinical outcomes. Use of the tool lead to better outcomes for young people after renal transplant [21] and was associated with a lower number of emergency room visits in young people with type 1 diabetes [29]. One quantitative controlled study did not find any significant short-term effects of the SGU-E on different outcomes, such as communication or self-management. However, the authors mention that this could be due to the lack of power of the study [3]. Finally, van Staa et al. [6] emphasized that despite an increase in discussions of non-medical topics, gaps between how important topics were rated by adolescents and how often these were discussed were still existent. They conclude that there is ample room for improvement in the application of individual transition plans.

8.8.1   Recommendations

1. Individual transition plans like the SGU and RSG are useful in practice, but it is recommended to tailor use of such tools, i.e. to select the right tool for the right person. There are for instance Easy Read versions for people with mild intellectual disabilities.

2. Professionals might benefit from proper guidance when implementing SGU or RSG to have a clear view on ownership of the tool and to prevent hesitation in discussing topics with young people. For both the SGU and the RSG there is an e-learning (in Dutch) available for professionals (https://www.free-learning.nl/modules/groei-wijzer-in-de-revalidatie/start.html and https://www.free-learning.nl/modules/readysteadygo/start.html). It is recommended that the whole healthcare team together works on an implementation plan before starting to work with either tool. Questions they should address in such a plan are for instance:
   (a) Who of the team will work with the tool?
   (b) When and how often will the tool be used?
   (c) Will the separate lists for parents also be used?
   (d) How can the tool be provided to young people and their parents? (On paper or digital)
   (e) How will action plans or agreements be documented and by whom?
   (f) How will results be shared among the team members; also during transfer to adult care?
   (g) Who will use the tool in adult care?
3. Good documentation of the process is important for the tools to be useful. It is recommended that teams develop a standardized way of documentation to be implemented in the electronic health record.
4. Finally, the paper form of the tools is time-consuming and brings logistic problems. Therefore, the integration of the SGU and RSG in electronic platforms used in healthcare is recommended. In the Netherlands for example, both tools are implemented in KLIK PROfile, which is an effective web-based application for the use of patient reported outcomes and experiences for monitoring [24, 30, 31].

8.9   Conclusion

Individual transition plans such as the SGU and RSG are useful tools to open up discussions about developmental tasks and challenges of young people with chronic conditions during healthcare consultations. Since these tasks and challenges are similar across conditions, the use of such generic tools seems appropriate. Young people, their parents and healthcare professionals all value the use of the tools and feel that it helps young people to become independent and to prepare for the future. They particularly appreciate the attention for generic developmental challenges. Furthermore it increases awareness and provides guidelines for all involved parties. Yet, effects on autonomy development are not underlined by effect studies yet. Also, the use of tools like the SGU and RSG requires flexibility and tailoring in clinical practice. However, attention for autonomy development is part of developmentally appropriate healthcare for young people and this is precisely what tools as the SGU and RSG foster.

References

1. Binks JA, Barden WS, Burke TA, Young NL. What do we really know about the transition to adult-centered health care? A focus on cerebral palsy and spina bifida. Arch Phys Med Rehabil. 2007;88(8):1064–73. https://doi.org/10.1016/j.apmr.2007.04.018.
2. Sawyer SM, Drew S, Yeo MS, Britto MT. Adolescents with a chronic condition: challenges living, challenges treating. Lancet. 2007;369(9571):1481–9. https://doi.org/10.1016/S0140-6736(07)60370-5.
3. Hilberink SR, van Ool M, van der Stege HA, van Vliet MC, van Heijningen-Tousain HJM, de Louw AJA, van Staa AL. Skills for growing up-epilepsy: an exploratory mixed methods study into a communication tool to promote autonomy and empowerment of youth with epilepsy. Epilepsy Behav. 2018;86:116–23. https://doi.org/10.1016/j.yebeh.2018.05.040.
4. Peeters MAC, Hilberink SR, van Staa AL. The road to independence: lived experiences of youth with chronic conditions and their parents compared. J Pediatr Rehabil Med. 2014;7(1):33–42. https://doi.org/10.3233/PRM-140272.
5. Betz CL, Lobo ML, Nehring WM, Bui K. Voices not heard: a systematic review of adolescents' and emerging adults' perspectives of health care transition. Nurs Outlook. 2013;61(5):311–36. https://doi.org/10.1016/j.outlook.2013.01.008.
6. van Staa AL, Sattoe JNT, Strating MM. Experiences with and outcomes of two interventions to maximize engagement of chronically ill adolescents during hospital consultations: a mixed methods study. J Pediatr Nurs. 2015;30(5):757–75. https://doi.org/10.1016/j.pedn.2015.05.028.
7. Ferris ME, Ferris MT, Okumura MJ, Cohen SE, Hooper SR. Health care transition preparation in youth with chronic conditions: working towards translational evidence with a patient perspective. J Pediatr Rehabil Med. 2015;8(1):31–7. https://doi.org/10.3233/PRM-150316.
8. Reiss JG, Gibson RW, Walker LR. Health care transition: youth, family, and provider perspectives. Pediatrics. 2005;115(1):112–20. https://doi.org/10.1542/peds.2004-1321.
9. Wood DL, Sawicki GS, Miller MD, Smotherman C, Lukens-Bull K, Livingood WC, Ferris M, Kraemer DF. The Transition Readiness Assessment Questionnaire (TRAQ): its factor structure, reliability, and validity. Acad Pediatr. 2014;14(4):415–22. https://doi.org/10.1016/j.jacap.2014.03.008.
10. Deci EL, Ryan RM. The "what" and "why" of goal pursuits: human needs and the self-determination of behavior. Psychol Inq. 2000;11(4):227–68. https://doi.org/10.1207/S15327965PLI1104_01.
11. Ryan RM, Deci EL. The darker and brighter sides of human existence: basic psychological needs as a unifying concept. Psychol Inq. 2000;11(4):319–38. https://doi.org/10.1207/S15327965PLI1104_03.
12. Chen B, Vansteenkiste M, Beyers W, Boone L, Deci EL, Van der Kaap-Deeder J, Duriez B, Lens W, Matos L, Mouratidis A, Ryan RM, Sheldon KM, Soenens B, Van Petegem S, Verstuyf J. Basic psychological need satisfaction, need frustration, and need strength across four cultures. Motiv Emot. 2015;39(2):216–36. https://doi.org/10.1007/s11031-014-9450-1.
13. Cardol M, De Jong BA, Ward CD. On autonomy and participation in rehabilitation. Disabil Rehabil. 2002;24(18):970–4. https://doi.org/10.1080/09638280210151996.
14. Maslow GR, Chung RJ. Systematic review of positive youth development programs for adolescents with chronic illness. Pediatrics. 2013;131(5):e1605–18. https://doi.org/10.1542/peds.2012-1615.
15. Gall C, Kingsnorth S, Healy H. Growing up ready: a shared management approach. Phys Occup Ther Pediatr. 2006;26(4):47–62. https://doi.org/10.1080/J006v26n04_04.
16. Hilberink SR, Grootoonk A, Ketelaar M, Vos I, Cornet L, Roebroeck ME. Focus on autonomy: using 'Skills for Growing Up' in pediatric rehabilitation care. J Pediatr Rehabil Med. 2020;13:161. https://doi.org/10.3233/PRM-190618.
17. Maathuis CGB, Vos I, Roebroeck ME, Hilberink SR. Een instrument om vaardigheden voor zelfstandigheid te vergroten. De Groei-wijzer [An instrument to improve skills for indepen-

dence. The Skills for Growing Up]. Nederlands Tijdschrift voor Revalidatiegeneeskunde. 2012;3:115–9.

18. Sattoe JNT, Hilberink SR, Peeters MA, van Staa AL. 'Skills for growing up': supporting autonomy in young people with kidney disease. J Ren Care. 2014;40(2):131–9. https://doi.org/10.1002/jorc.12046.

19. Holland Bloorview Kids Rehabilitation Hospital. Guidelines for service providers – supporting youth & families in using the skills for growing up checklists. Toronto, ON: Holland Bloorview Kids Rehabilitation Hospital; 2007.

20. McDonagh JE, Southwood TR, Shaw KL. Growing up and moving on in rheumatology: development and preliminary evaluation of a transitional care programme for a multicentre cohort of adolescents with juvenile idiopathic arthritis. J Child Health Care. 2006;10(1):22–42. https://doi.org/10.1177/1367493506060203.

21. Connett GJ, Nagra A. Ready, steady, go - achieving successful transition in cystic fibrosis. Paediatr Respir Rev. 2018;27:13–5. https://doi.org/10.1016/j.prrv.2018.05.007.

22. Nagra A, McGinnity PM, Davis N, Salmon AP. Implementing transition: ready steady go. Archiv Dis Childhood Educ Pract. 2015;100(6):313–20. https://doi.org/10.1136/archdischild-2014-307423.

23. Nagra A. Ready steady go: easy read. Southampton: Southampton Children's Hospital; 2019. https://www.uhs.nhs.uk/OurServices/Childhealth/TransitiontoadultcareReadySteadyGo/Ready-Steady-Go-Easy-read.aspx.

24. Zalmijn RA, Vreugdenhil HIJ, van Oers HA, McDonald-ten Thij C, Buizer AI. E-Health: Met de Groei-wijzer digitaal 'KLIKken' op weg naar zelfstandigheid [E-health: with the skills for growing up digitally 'CLICKing' towards independence]. Nederlands Tijdschrift voor Revalidatiegeneeskunde. 2020;42(2):44–6.

25. van der Slikke M, Bronner M, van Staa AL. Klaar voor de overstap met Ready Steady Go. [Ready to transfer with ready steady go]. Magazine Kinderverpleegkunde [Mag Paediat Nurs]. 2018;24(1):16–8.

26. McDonald C. Introduction to the transition programme Ready Steady Go for adolescents with spina bifida: usability and satisfaction (Master's thesis). Amsterdam: Inholland University; 2019.

27. van Staa AL, van der Stege HA, Hilberink SR, van Vliet MC, van Heijningen-Tousain HJM, et al. Ontwikkeling, test, brede implementatie en evaluatie van de Epilepsie Groei-wijzer voor kinderen/jongeren met epilepsie met en zonder licht verstandelijke beperkingen [Development, testing, broad implementation and evaluation of the skills for growing up - epilepsy for children/young people with epilepsy with and without mild intellectual disabilities]. Rotterdam: Rotterdam University of Applied Sciences; 2017.

28. VRA, Netherlands Society of Rehabilitation Medicine. Spastic cerebral palsy in children. Treatment guideline. Utrecht: Netherlands Society of Rehabilitation Medicine; 2015. https://richtlijnendatabase.nl/richtlijn/spastische_cerebrale_parese_bij_kinderen/spastische_cerebrale_parese_-_startpagina.html#verantwoording.

29. Cable L, Davis N. Service evaluation of the 'Ready Steady Go' transition programme in type 1 diabetes in Southampton. Endoc Abst. 2015;39:EP37. https://doi.org/10.1530/endoabs.39.EP37.

30. Haverman L, Engelen V, van Rossum MA, Heymans HS, Grootenhuis MA. Monitoring health-related quality of life in paediatric practice: development of an innovative web-based application. BMC Pediatr. 2011;11(1):3. https://doi.org/10.1186/1471-2431-11-3.

31. Haverman L, van Rossum MA, van Veenendaal M, van den Berg JM, Dolman KM, Swart J, Kuijpers TW, Grootenhuis MA. Effectiveness of a web-based application to monitor health-related quality of life. Pediatrics. 2013;131(2):e533–43. https://doi.org/10.1542/peds.2012-0958.